# RECLAIMING BIRTH:
History and Heroines of American Childbirth Reform

# RECLAIMING BIRTH:

## History and Heroines
## of American Childbirth Reform

by Margot Edwards and Mary Waldorf

THE CROSSING PRESS/Trumansburg, New York 14886

Permission to reprint from the following publications is gratefully acknowledged:

THE TENDER GIFT: BREASTFEEDING by Dana Raphael (New York, Prentice Hall, 1973) by consent of the author

BIRTH CONTROL AND CONTROLLING BIRTH edited by Helen B. Holmes et al. (Clifton, N.J., The Humana Press, 1980)

"Gerda Lerner on the Future of Our Past" by Catherine R. Stimson in MS., September, 1981

Library of Congress Cataloging in Publication Data

Edwards, Margot.
   Reclaiming birth.

   Includes bibliographical references and index.
   1. Childbirth—United States—History. 2. Childbirth—
Study and teaching—United States—History. 3. Health
reformers—United States. I. Waldorf, Mary. II. Title.
RG652.E38   1984          618.2          84-1859
ISBN 0-89594-129-5
ISBN 0-89594-128-7 (pbk.)

# ACKNOWLEDGMENTS

We are deeply grateful to family and friends who supported our efforts during this five-year project. Special gratitude goes to John Neighbours who guided us through the mysteries of the word processor. We thank David Edwards who proofread and renewed tired spirits, and Penny Simkin, Celeste McLeod, Ruth Wilf, Sheryle Paukert, Gay Courter, Dan Edwards, and Elizabeth Waldorf, all of whom read sections of the manuscript and offered useful criticism when we needed it most. For helping us with research and sharing special recollections, we thank Margaret Gamper, Virginia Larson, M.D., Helen Wessel, Edith Patton, Lynn Moen, Penny Simkin, Arnold Manor, M.D., Moses Greenfield, Madeleine Shearer and Carole Erickson. Norma Swenson and Lynn Moen offered us early and continuing encouragement for which we are very grateful. We appreciate also Ruth Gottstein's interest in the manuscript. Others who contributed to the work in various ways include Tessa Eckman, Leena Valvanne, Rosemary Fost, India Harrison, Gail Brewer, Diane Reed and many counselors and childbirth educators from women's groups all over the United States; in particular, the Childbirth Education League of the Monterey Peninsula. Thanks go to Niles Newton and the founding mothers of La Leche League International who met with us in Chicago and to all the featured women: Margaret Gamper, Elisabeth Bing, Lester Hazell, Niles Newton, Doris Haire, Sheila Kitzinger, and Raven Lang, whose willingness to share their lives made this book possible. We have been fortunate in working with a talented and enthusiastic editor, Andrea Fleck Clardy of The Crossing Press.

*Margot Edwards and Mary Waldorf, Monterey, California, December 1983.*

# CONTENTS

INTRODUCTION: Childbirth, the Eye of the Needle     vii

CHAPTER ONE:
NATURAL AND UNNATURAL—CHILDBIRTH 1930–1950     1

    Childbirth as Pathology     4
    Chicago Maternity Center     6
    Frontier Nursing Service     10
    Maternity Center Association of New York     12
    Grantly Dick-Read: Prophet of Reclaiming Birth     14
    *Margaret Gamper: Pioneer Childbirth Educator     18

CHAPTER TWO: STIRRINGS OF PROTEST 1950–1970     29

    *Elisabeth Bing and the Lamaze Solution     33
    The Fight over Natural Childbirth     40
    Marjorie Karmel     42
    ASPO—The American Society for Psychoprophylaxis
       in Obstetrics     48
    Cruelty on the Maternity Wards     54
    *Lester Hazell: Getting What You Want with ICEA     57

CHAPTER THREE: DECLINE AND RESURRECTION OF
BREAST FEEDING 1900–PRESENT     69

    Summer Illness     69
    Reign of the Experts and Loss of
       Maternal Confidence 1900–1960     75
    *Niles Newton: A Scientist Attacks
       Medical Myths on Nursing     78
    La Leche League: Our Lady of Bountiful Milk
       and Easy Delivery     87

Breastfeeding and Sex                                                    90
Breastfeeding and Working Mothers                                        95
Radicals Rise from the Ranks of the LLLI                                 97

CHAPTER FOUR:
SAGA OF OBSTETRICAL TECHNOLOGY                                          100

*Doris Haire: Lobbyist                                                  109
Banta and Thacker Question Effectiveness of EFM                         117
Brackbill: Long-term Effects of O.B. Drugs                              121
Marieskind: Cesarean, The Ultimate O.B. Technology                     123
Liebeskind: Seeing with Sound, Its Safety in Obstetrics                127
Opposition to High Tech Childbirth in England                          132
*Sheila Kitzinger: The Splendid Ritual                                 133
The Politics of Episiotomy                                             142

CHAPTER FIVE: THE MIDWIFE QUESTION                                     146

Old and New-Age Midwives                                               146
*Raven Lang: Lay Midwife                                               156
Midwife Arrests in California 1974–1982                                164
Aftermath of Midwife Arrests                                           174
Nashville Story                                                         179
Birthing Centers in and out of Hospital                                182

CONCLUSION: Transforming Consciousness                                 189

Notes                                                                  197
Index                                                                  215

*Featured women.

# INTRODUCTION

> Childbirth is the eye of the needle through which all of society passes under medicine's direction.
>
> *Norma Swenson*[1]

This book grew out of a beginning friendship between the authors. Sharing our past histories, we discovered common ground in lingering disappointment with our own first experiences in giving birth. From that discovery came the urge to take some sort of action. At first we intended simply to record the lives of seven contemporary women, major activists in education and reform whose work had been aimed at reclaiming birth for the birthing woman.

Margot, a childbirth educator and member of the reform movement, had met all the women at one time or another at conferences and during meetings of committees and editorial boards. They were all well-known as innovators and teachers in the childbirth field. However, like their forerunners in the profession, they seemed in danger of slipping out of history. Even in the woman's world of birthing babies, innovation and reform have long been dominated by the names of male obstetricians, and methods originated or developed by nurses, physical therapists, or midwives, if they survive at all, are known by the name of whichever medical man made them famous. We say "Lamaze method" without reference to Mme. Cohen who translated his Pavlovian ideas into lessons for pregnant women; we speak of Read as the founder of natural childbirth, but no one remembers Dr. Mary Ries Melendy who proposed just the same relationship between fear and pain in 1913; few are aware of Helen Heardman, the English physical therapist who developed the essential exercises associated with the Read method and introduced them to Americans at Grace-New Haven Hospital. We hoped to rectify some of those omissions, at least as far as they have occurred in the last fifty years when the major push for reform and education has taken place.

This was an era of great change in birth practices. Hospitalization became almost universal for American women, and from the beginning, intervention was part of hospital routine. Among obstetricians, the argument was usually over which drugs and which instruments, and not whether to use them at all. The history of obstetrics has been, in fact, the history of increasingly sophisticated intervention. These seven women and all others in the reform movement have in one way or another continued to question the nature of that intervention.

When Margaret Gamper, eldest of the seven, began to coach laboring women in 1946, the majority of deliveries were performed on mothers rendered unconscious or nearly so with a variety of drugs. Very few professionals shared Margaret's hope that Read methods of controlling pain would provide an alternative. Fewer still, and probably among them no other nurses, were willing to stake an independent career on that faith, as she did. As a young woman she had run away from home to become a nurse. On the verge of middle age, she displayed similar spirit in striking out on her own as a childbirth educator, an endeavor she still conducts well into her eighth decade.

Showing the same radical independence in the seventies, Californian Raven Lang came to the art and skill of midwifery through her own devices, an empiric committed to the rights of women to take up the skills they need in caring for one another. She is known as a mythmaker, an almost legendary figure among the midwives, and is the veteran of several battles with traditional authority that reopened the old and bitter debate about midwifery and its right to exist.

Elisabeth Bing, born into a cosmopolitan European culture that vanished in the Second World War, encountered Read's work in London about the same time as did Margaret Gamper in Chicago. Both women were established as health professionals before becoming involved in labor coaching. Each, following years of longing and grief over infertility, bore a child when she was almost forty. When her son arrived, Elisabeth had already been teaching Read methods in New York City for several years and continued to do so until 1959 when she met Marjorie Karmel who had had a baby under the care of the controversial Fernand Lamaze in Paris. Believing the new method of active participation was more suitable to American women, Elisabeth shifted to Lamaze. The best known of American childbirth educators, she was the chief founder of an organization that made "Lamaze" a household word and very nearly synonymous with prepared childbirth in the United States.

Doris Haire, like Lester Hazell, came into the reform movement through volunteer parent groups, but she eventually grew impatient with attempts to alter institutions by educating parents and took more direct action. Since the mid-seventies, she has been regularly marching into what she calls the "lions' dens" of Washington where representatives of industry, medicine and government debate regulations that directly affect obstetrical practice. Undaunted by what is often a chilly welcome, she has lobbied vigorously in cooperation with the National Women's Health Network for the rights of pregnant women and their infants.

Niles Newton's initiation into the field took place while she was nursing her second baby in 1947. As an academic psychologist, she was struck by the lack of scientific data on breastfeeding. Using herself and her infant daughter for experiments, Niles made observations that revealed why so few women could nurse their babies. Radicalized by the circumstances surrounding the birth of her third child, she embarked on more research, published more scientific papers, and ultimately came to question the entire set of assumptions which govern health practices for women.

This larger view marks much of the work of the two remaining women, both anthropologists as well as birth educators. Lester Hazell, sometimes called the philosopher of childbirth reform, began coaching other women in labor following a grievous experience in the birth of her first child. One of the earliest and most eloquent spokespersons for the rights of parents, she developed a concept of birth as both a passage and a transcendent experience where "for a moment one shares the universe."[2] Sheila Kitzinger, the Oxford-educated social anthropologist and energetic leader of British reform, has observed birth in many different cultures. Like Lester, she sees every birth as a symbolic event, signifying hope and continuation for the life of a people. The mother of five daughters all born at home, Sheila developed her own method, strongly influenced by the belief that giving birth is a sexual act, a theory also supported by the work of Niles Newton.

Much of our information on the women was gained from personal interviews that revealed subjective experiences as well as work records. We decided to include both, feeling that details in the lives of women struggling to become themselves are a vital part of womens' history. The network of public events added another dimension. In order to present the women's lives in the perspective of their contributions to childbirth education, we had to provide some account of allied stories, such as the midwife trials, the long-running conflicts over drugged labor and natural childbirth, and the politics of obstetrical hardware. In addition to professional journals and histories, we searched newspapers and back issues of women's magazines like *Ladies' Home Journal* and *Redbook* where we found more evidence of a continuing struggle over who was to control the process of childbearing in America. Physicians, social scientists, novelists, and journalists argued the subject in the pages of these magazines. Occasionally space was given to experiences of everyday women, most stunningly in a 1958 *Ladies' Home Journal* series titled "Cruelty on the Maternity Wards."

During the extended period of research, our project grew, and what began as a collection of lives became a history of American childbirth during the past half century with some developments from earlier times. In terms of her contribution to childbirth reform, each woman seemed to belong to a particular cluster of historical events. Margaret Gamper emerges most sharply through the first struggles for reform, heralded by Read in England. The life of Doris Haire is inextricable from an account of the current explosion of technology. Raven Lang's life is embedded in the decline of midwifery and its present resurrection. Elisabeth Bing's influence grew with the Lamaze revolution. Niles Newton's work gave support to the founding mothers of La Leche League, while Lester Hazell is known primarily through the growth of the National Association of Parents and Professionals for Safe Alternatives in Childbirth. Sheila Kitzinger, prime leader of British resistance to imported high-tech obstetrics, is also known for her evaluation of birth rituals old and new.

Each of these women emerged from a different milieu and traveled a slightly different path formed by the circumstances of her private life and the public events of a particular time. Yet in the original definition of the term 'midwife,' they all came to stand before the laboring woman with a common ideal: that she would pass through this profound experience with awareness of what was happening in her body, with some control over how others dealt with it, and with a degree of choice in how and where the experience was to take place.

We took note of feminist historian Gerda Lerner's theory that the ordinary experience of family life, including caring for the old, the ailing, and the young, is largely undertaken by women whether they have borne children or not, and involves an aspect of life that is essential to all humankind, be they men, women, or children. Deprived of it, we are in danger of becoming monstrous beings capable of "pursuing possibility without restraint . . . of alienating the individual without restraint . . . of dividing the work of the world in such a way that some think and others act, that some are occupied with ordering the world and others with housekeeping it . . . "[3]

The women we have featured and many others working in childbirth reform are involved in a struggle to dignify the ordinary experience of women as they become mothers, thus contributing to the salvation of life's essential human quality. And we hope also, in recounting their lives against a context of childbirth history, that we have made a contribution to the yet untold story of female culture, uncovering a small part of what Adrienne Rich called the "immense half-buried mosaic in the shape of a woman's face."[4]

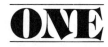

# ONE

# Natural and Unnatural-Childbirth 1930-1950

In my opinion, no woman whether intelligent or unintelligent, modern or old-fashioned, wants the birth of a baby a blank in her memory. Certainly, none will wish to be relieved of pain at the risk of harm to the baby.[1]

This statement and others by Gertrude Nielsen, an Oklahoma City physician and mother, caused an uproar in the 1936 American Medical Association symposium on obstetrics. The ensuing controversy hit the front page of *The New York Times* under the headline, "Doctors Assail Twilight Birth as Perilous to Mother and Child." Dr. Nielsen, running counter to a contemporary enthusiasm for totally anesthetized deliveries, had been preceded on the AMA rostrum by three groups of doctors extolling their successes in over seven thousand drugged births. Nevertheless, she declared her belief that the high maternal death rate (then about six per thousand births) was in large part a result of the use of analgesics. "An analgesic that is perfectly safe for mother and child has not been discovered," she said. Anything that deadened sensation distorted natural processes and depressed respiratory functions in the infant.

Nielsen, the mother of three children born without the use of drugs, said she favored a more natural course in labor. Women suffered pain largely because they were filled with fear, a fear that had been increased by "irresponsible allusions to the dangers of childbirth and by sensational magazine articles which have gone so far as to advocate cesarean section as the only humane method of delivery."[2] *The Times* reporter further attributed to her the assertion that doctors could allay a woman's fear by explaining that the pain lay largely in the minds of magazine writers. If doctors minimized the fear of pain, they might preserve the natural elation that belongs to birth, whereas a woman deprived of the experience through drugs could suffer mental anguish as a result. Psychoanalyses, she was reported to have said, had shown that many nervous disorders of women could be traced to the psychic injuries of unnatural birth.

At a time when many women felt that being modern and independent included freedom from the childbed suffering of their mothers, Dr. Nielsen's attack seemed like reactionary nonsense in the view of most obstetricians. Still, she had a few supporters at the symposium. One physician acknowledged she had merely spoken aloud what many felt but dared not mention. Another, Joseph B. DeLee, the chief proponent of childbirth as pathological, agreed that labor pain was largely psychological and that the mother's mental condition would affect those muscles engaged in expelling the infant. Another doctor remarked that American obstetrics was becoming a competitive practice to please American women in accordance with what they read in lay magazines.[3]

At the height of the debate, Dr. Rudolph Holmes of Chicago made a dramatic confession. He was responsible, he said, for introducing "twilight sleep" (scopolamine and morphine) to American labor rooms. "I didn't know what I was doing. I have found out since. . . . We must protest vigorously against making the human mother an animated mass without any mentality."[4]

In the protests that followed *The Times* story, none of the questions about the safety of drugs for birth were dealt with, nor was Holmes' confession. The response focused on what appeared to be Nielsen's moral stance in favor of pain. In letters to the editor, women sputtered with fury at being told their pains were wrought by journalists, as if they hadn't the wit to know whether they were in actual agony or not. "A woman who has given birth has nothing to fear from hell," one wrote. Another likened labor pain to a crucifixion, saying she had felt like a wounded animal trapped in a jungle. A reader warned that there was a "purgatory waiting for doctors indifferent to the agony of childbirth." Another asked caustically whether Queen Victoria had read magazine articles prior to her daring request for chloroform at the birth of her seventh child in 1850.[5] Several readers were indignant at Nielsen's suggestion that missing the first few moments of her child's life might affect a mother's relationship with the child, a concept that became dogma forty years later. In 1936, the notion was dismissed as a relic of the benighted past.

Bruce and Beatrice Gould, editors of the influential *Ladies' Home Journal* which set standards of taste and fashion, manners and ethics for thousands of American women, were dismayed by Nielsen's reported belief that pain was good for the spirit. That was similar, they wrote, to a surgeon's holding back the chloroform for an amputation on the grounds of spiritual improvement for the patient.[6]

The magazine *Nation* editorialized with even greater scorn. Nielsen's ideas were apparently derived from the Biblical condemnation of women to pain in labor, a notion long discarded by modern scientific culture. The editors charged that, according to Nielsen's theory, doctors who had formerly offended God by relieving pain were now offending Freud. They consulted their own expert, a psychoanalyst trained by the great man himself. He called the notion that drugged childbirth might harm a woman's psyche "vicious and sadistic nonsense." According to the editorial, he also remarked that, "since the complex and nerve-wracking life of civilization (not the magazine writers) has interfered with the automatic nature of the child-bearing process, the least civilization can do for the woman in childbirth is to find means to alleviate the agony for which it is largely responsible."[7]

In a letter, Nielsen protested vigorously against this assessment of her stand, adding, "I am not unmindful of the progress made in this direction (alleviation of pain) by the use of analgesics, but insist that efforts should also be made to counteract the detrimental influences of civilization by proper prenatal education and suitable obstetrical management. . . . As the process by which childbirth has been distorted becomes better understood, an increasing number of women may be enabled to experience easy, natural childbirth without excessive use of drugs."[8]

However, at that time very few people questioned the belief that progress had somehow destroyed women's ability to give birth unless aided by men and their instruments. And those few often went unheard. Gena Corea uncovered the history of one critic,

Dorothy Reed Mendenhall, a woman doctor who began to question American obstetrics after she lost her first-born at the hands of the "best doctor" in her town. He injured her so badly in performing a version (turning the fetus in the uterus) and in delivery that another physician examining her later said, "It was a miracle you survived such obstetrics."[9]

As a researcher for the Children's Bureau, a government agency promoting maternal-infant welfare, Mendenhall discovered in 1925 that more than three times as many women died during childbirth in Washington D.C. hospitals as those who gave birth at home. The following year she observed birth practices in Denmark, a country where mortality rates for both mothers and infants were much lower than in the U.S. The difference in management was that the Danes favored non-interference, employing midwives for 85 percent of their deliveries. Mendenhall's report was generally ignored or disparaged by physicians, as were many of the Bureau's recommendations for reform, and her work slipped out of sight. Corea recorded a poignant conclusion taken from Mendenhall's private papers: "Most of my work came out of my agony and grief. All the writing and teaching on safe maternity I have thought of as a memorial to Margaret, my first child and only girl."[10]

## Childbirth as Pathology

The experiences and opinions of the two women, despite the fact that both were physicians, were disregarded by most of the members of their speciality where obstetricians, overwhelmingly male, had long assumed authority in describing how the birth process felt for both mother and child. One of the most influential of that period, Joseph B. DeLee painted a picture of birth as a horrifying ordeal for the participants, requiring the aid of surgical intervention. He had presented this view in an influential paper offered to the AMA convention in 1920. Initially controversial and even criticized as advocating "meddlesome midwifery," it was accepted within a few years by all but a handful of U.S. obstetricians.[11] (Ironically, DeLee was also the founder of the Chicago Maternity Center, whose record of low-technology birth care stands in such contrast to his view of the dangers of giving birth.)

DeLee illustrated his theory with harsh images. Birth for the infant, he said, was equivalent to having one's head squeezed in a slowly closing door, a description similar to Frederick Leboyer's of the innocent fetus forced out of the womb by a monstrous mother who then compounded the cruelty by obstructing escape from her imprisoning body.[12] DeLee believed the repeated thrusts down the birth canal, head pounding against the rigid perineum, were in some cases responsible for brain damage, epilepsy, and cerebral palsy.

He differed from Leboyer in observing that mothers suffered as well, seldom escaping injury in an ordeal as brutal as having a pitchfork driven through her perineum. "So frequent are these bad effects that I have often wondered whether Nature did not deliberately intend women to be used up in the process of reproduction in a manner analogous to that of the salmon which dies after spawning."[13]

His remedy was to sedate the women during the first stages of labor, use ether during the second, make a cut of several inches to enlarge the vaginal opening and then lift the fetus out with forceps. Afterward, ergot would be administered to contract the uterus, followed by mechanical removal of the placenta and suturing of the incision. Women would thereby be restored to what he called "virginal conditions" and the infant saved from the worst of the torture.

The initial objections from within the profession were not to his evaluation of birth as disease but to his remedy. At that time, DeLee's main rival for dominance in obstetrics was John Whitridge Williams, head of obstetrics at Johns Hopkins and, like DeLee, author of a textbook in the field. He declared that if DeLee's procedures were generally adopted, the results for women would be worse than if they had been attended by midwives, a profession thoroughly discredited by physicians. DeLee conceded the operation was not justifiable unless undertaken by an expert. However, these reservations were swept away in the enthusiastic acceptance of birth as a pathological event requiring the skills of a trained interventionist. The use of forceps and episiotomy became so routine in the sixty years following DeLee's presentation that hardly anyone in the profession bothered to wonder why they were instituted in the first place. (Dr. David Banta's studies on episiotomy in 1981 are a rare exception. See Chapter Four.)

There is no doubt that doctors of the time were seeing a great many tears and injuries during birth, which DeLee attributed to pathology inherent in the process. But, as Richard and Dorothy Wertz pointed out in their history of childbirth, these complications may also have come from the almost universal requirement that hospital deliveries take place while the woman lay flat on her back with her legs spread and held aloft in stirrups (the lithotomy position considered by reformers one of the worst for giving birth).[14]

DeLee's major experience had come from attending the labors of poor women in the Chicago slums. Unlike many of his colleagues, he was born in modest circumstances, one of ten children in an immigrant Polish-Jewish family. Perhaps because of his background, he was concerned with the poverty-stricken women he delivered while interning at Cook County Hospital. DeLee decided to open a clinic for these women with a twofold purpose: the first was to provide them with free or low-cost care, and the second was to provide teaching material for his obstetrical students. In the early days, he paid women a quarter each to allow him to deliver them.

Funded by contributions from friends and the Young Men's Hebrew Association, DeLee's Maxwell Street Dispensary opened in four rooms of a tenement building. At first, DeLee and his students attended all women at home, but later small maternity hospitals were set up in association with the dispensary. Work continued under his leadership until 1932 when he left to become chief of obstetrics at a vast new hospital, Chicago Lying-In. Unwilling to let the Maxwell Street Dispensary die, he arranged financial support, and the old dispensary became the Chicago Maternity Center. It grew into one of the rare facilities where emphasis on a more natural course prevailed, running counter to dominant trends in twentieth century obstetrics, particularly those of its founder.

## The Chicago Maternity Center

Housed in the original building at the corner of Newberry and Maxwell Streets, the Center began functioning in 1932, primarily as a home birth service under the directorship of a remarkable woman, Beatrice Tucker, who had just finished a residency at Chicago Lying-In. Some four years later, Paul De Kruif, biologist and popular medical writer, focused on the Center in a series of articles for *Ladies' Home Journal*, titled "Why Should Mothers Die?" De Kruif began by noting that while death rates from diseases such as tuberculosis had fallen dramatically in the first third of the century, women were dying in childbirth at much the same rate as they had before science made such great strides. In the past twenty-five years, he wrote, 375,000 women died as a result of pregnancy and childbirth, more than all the men killed in all the nation's wars since the Declaration of Independence. Strangely, the poor, malnourished and ill-housed women of Chicago who were attended by Dr. Tucker and the Maternity Center staff, died far less often in childbirth. De Kruif wondered why.

Four lengthy articles, published through the spring of 1936, were meant as an answer to that question, an answer that could be applied elsewhere to alleviate the high death rate among American mothers, long ignored by the medical profession. Obstetrics had always been considered a third-rate speciality, something any dolt could manage, and certainly far from the exciting frontier of scientific medicine. De Kruif confessed that he, too, had formerly viewed the profession of baby-bringing with contempt. Now, having spent hours at the Chicago Maternity Center in the company of its "young death fighters" and deeply impressed by the former director and "master birth-helper," DeLee, he saw his error. "I understand now that there is no speciality in the whole art and science of doctoring that demands such a complicated thorough knowledge of diagnosis, of microbe hunting, of psychology, of the art of giving anesthetics, and of the boldest and most subtle wielding of the surgeon's knife."[15]

This romanticized view of the savior-scientist shepherding the little human through the most dangerous journey of its existence was to prevail. The odd aspect is that De Kruif chose to illustrate his view with the Chicago Maternity Center. The Center, which stood in the heart of what De Kruif called one of Chicago's ugliest slums, functioned from the beginning as a home birth service. The cries of the vendors and the quacking and squawking of doomed poultry at nearby Maxwell Market competed with the constant activity at the clinic with pregnant women going to and fro, the obstetrical team departing hurriedly or returning after a delivery, and with the activities of staff members who often lived at the Center, sleeping in basement rooms as Dr. Tucker did for years. When a telephone call announced that a patient had gone into labor, a team of midwives, nurses, and student doctors departed by streetcar to attend her, often in tenement rooms or cottages that lacked indoor plumbing and sometimes even floors.

In these difficult circumstances the CMC people were determined to prevent maternal death, especially that caused by childbed fever (puerperal sepsis), the disease that continued to kill newly-delivered women until the late thirties. The source of the poisoning, hemolytic streptococcus, had been suspected since the Hungarian Ignatz

Semmelweis broke his career and sanity in the 1850s by trying to persuade his fellow doctors that they themselves were carrying the deadly germs as they moved from diseased women to well ones without washing their hands or changing clothes. A decade earlier an American doctor, Oliver Wendell Holmes, had provoked great indignation by proposing the same theory. One colleague responded that Holmes' accusation that doctors were carrying the disease could not be correct since doctors were gentlemen and gentlemen had clean hands.[16] However, following Lister's success in preventing wound infections with carbolic acid in the 1860s, American doctors slowly began to accept the need for antiseptic conditions. (It was not until the late 1930s that the virulence of childbed fever was reduced by a number of factors, notably the discovery of antibiotics.)

The Maternity Center staff members were fanatic in their attention to cleanliness in themselves and to producing antiseptic conditions, if at all possible, in the rooms where they delivered. In the first two years of the Center's existence, only thirteen mothers died, and of these thirteen, four deaths were from infection. In one case, before the team could reach the laboring woman, she was examined by "an old crone of a Mississippi granny" who touched her with unwashed hands, wrote De Kruif. Thereafter, Tucker required staff members to redouble their efforts in keeping clean. When De Kruif interviewed her in 1936, there had not been a single maternal death for two and a half years. He recorded an interesting conversation between the director and her assistant in response to his query: were their good statistics due to luck?

> "No—it may be the fact they have their babies in the homes, that's important," said the assistant director. The director bristled: "But we're not filthy, Benny!" "No, we're clean. We're the cleanest I've ever seen," he answered. "But even so, I could show you slips in technique in almost every mother delivered. No—it's the women's homes! They're probably immune from the bugs in their own homes! And we don't carry in any live virulent germs."[17]

In addition to their "austere fanatical cleanliness," De Kruif noted another probable reason for the low maternal death rate, and that was the Center's policy of allowing all babies to be born naturally and without operations, if that could be managed without harm to the mother. In view of this philosophy of non-interference, De Kruif's conclusion that the application of *more* expert interference was needed to prevent other mothers from death seems oddly askew. However, he was writing during a period when it was widely believed that science was on the verge of solving all humanity's ills, so what did not fit that vision might be noted but not taken seriously. For De Kruif, the student doctors at the Center were always "young death fighters," and their weapons were the skills of the microbe hunter, the anesthetist and the surgeon, gifts from what he called "the amazing new science of life's good morning."[18]

During her forty years as director of the Center, Beatrice Tucker must have altered her vision of perfect science as applied to birth. In 1973, during an exhausting and ultimately doomed battle to save CMC from closure by Northwestern University administrators, Dr. Tucker declared that she was committed to home births. "At home, of course, deliveries are by natural childbirth. We have more pain. But in a hospital the isolation is devastating. Both results are good. I believe a patient has a right to choose where she wants to have her baby."[19]

These statements are more startling when Tucker's training and background are considered. After receiving an M.D. and interning as the first woman at Evanston Hospital, she worked in a variety of settings. For several years she served the most deprived citizens of the city as physician to the Morals Court and Women's Department of the Chicago City Jail and as clinician in the Infant Welfare Clinic. Later she assisted a woman surgeon whose patients were affluent suburbanites. In 1929 she returned to an earlier interest in obstetrics and persuaded a reluctant DeLee to accept her as the first woman resident at Chicago Lying-In. "The training received under his direction permitted real competition for the first time in my experience with men specialists for coveted hospital appointments and other desirable affiliations."[20]

So here was a young doctor who had fought her way into a male specialty, trained at the hands of the architect of obstetrical intervention—a man who had proposed as early as 1913 that the "pathological dignity of obstetrics" be fully recognized.[21] Yet after four decades of serving Chicago's poor women in tenement rooms with limited equipment, Dr. Tucker was convinced that women could be delivered safely at home.

Although its patients were considered high risk during labor and delivery, the statistics on 150,000 Center births remained excellent; in fact, women delivering under CMC care were eight to ten times safer than those at Cook County Hospital.[22] Nevertheless, administrators of Northwestern University Medical School moved to destroy the CMC, one declaring that the kind of service it offered had "no place in the women's health care industry."[23] In a classic maneuver, they took over the Center, saying it was to be relocated in a new women's hospital. But once the administrators had control and were free from community protests, they abolished CMC entirely along with all home birth facilities.

At the time, in 1974, Dr. Tucker was seventy-five years old. Her remarkable accomplishment in directing a home birth service for poor women, largely Black and Hispanic, in one of the nation's most crowded urban areas is little known outside Chicago and seldom acknowledged by others in the field. A history of the speciality from colonial times to the present, published by the American College of Obstetricians and Gynecologists in 1980, covers the story of the Chicago Maternity Center from its inception to its demise, and celebrates DeLee as founder but never mentions Dr. Beatrice Tucker by name.[24]

## Frontier Nursing Service

The second low-technology maternal service with an enviable record of survival for mothers and infants was Mary Breckenridge's model of rural midwifery in the Kentucky Appalachians. Breckenridge, daughter of an affluent family with a tradition of social service, was widowed and then divorced while still a relatively young woman. Already trained as a nurse, she decided to spend the rest of her life providing medical care to the poor. After taking a course in public health nursing at Columbia, she worked for the American Committee for Relief in Belgium and France following World War I and later studied midwifery at the British Hospital for Mothers and Babies in London, achieving certification by the English Central Midwifery Board. By then she had conceived a plan for establishing a nursing service based on the practice of midwifery in her native Kentucky. A tour through the Scottish Highlands gave her an opportunity to see how decentralized health care could be managed in remote areas, and she came home in 1925 determined to use the same sort of system in Kentucky.

She chose an area of Leslie County dominated by a rugged stretch of the Appalachian Mountains where there were no roads and no railroad tracks. Everything that came into the isolated farms and mountain communities had to be brought on horseback or dragged by mule-drawn sled. Aside from attendance by granny midwives, professional health care was almost nonexistent.

With the aid of a newly organized Kentucky Committee for Mothers and Babies, Breckenridge set up a network of nurse midwives trained in Britain to serve a portion of the county, hoping eventually to expand the service to cover a thousand square miles. Each nurse was to live in a log or stone cabin in the center of her own district, serving all people within a five-mile radius. Her most important duty was to serve as a midwife offering care before, during and after birth to the mountain women. Secondly, she was to oversee the health of the infants and children. Finally, she was to offer preventive care and nursing to the general population as designated by the State Board of Health.

In 1926 the women set to work, led by Breckenridge herself. Traveling on horseback over rugged country, they delivered babies, kept watch on children, treated people for hookworm, chlorinated wells, and gave innoculations against typhoid and diphtheria. These nurse midwives shared the frontier life of those they served and followed the rule of their organization articulated by Breckenridge in 1928: "If a father can come for us, the nurse can go with him."[25]

Eunice Ernst, who came to the FNS as a young, traditionally trained nurse in the forties, dreamed of riding horses and doing public health nursing, not practicing midwifery. Her previous experience in obstetrics had largely been confined to keeping drugged mothers "up on the bed and down off the walls" during labor. She described her astonishment at witnessing her first home birth with a Frontier nurse midwife in attendance. "As I stood spellbound in my corner, I couldn't believe that a child had been born with so little fuss—with the mother in absolute control, with nurses who seemed to be able to speak with their eyes, teach with their hands and comfort with their presence."[26]

From its inception in 1925 to 1952, the FNS staff attended nine thousand births in which there were eleven maternal deaths. The national average of maternal mortality during those years was six times greater. Although obstetricians have been added to the regular staff for emergencies since 1952, nurse midwives still attend 90 percent of the births, and during this period there have been no maternal deaths. In 1932, Metropolitan Life reported on a study of the service and its first thousand births: "If such a service were available to women of the country generally there would be a saving of 10,000 mothers' lives each year in the United States, there would be 30,000 less stillbirths and 30,000 more children alive at the end of the first month of life. The study demonstrates that the first need today is to train a large body of nurse midwives, competent to carry out the routines which have been established in the FNS and other places where good obstetrical care is available."[27]

Although the FNS was seen as a model of service to remote areas and its midwives glorified as "angels on horseback," the example of what could be accomplished in home births attended by trained women was not taken seriously elsewhere in the U.S.. In the growing urban centers, women continued in greater and greater numbers to undergo birth in hospitals where pregnancy was treated as an illness.

## The Maternity Center Association of New York

An urban institution promoting non-intervention in birth was established somewhat earlier. This was the New York Maternity Center Association which grew out of philanthropic campaigns in the late nineteenth century to provide pure tuberculosis-free milk for the babies and toddlers of a largely immigrant population in New York City. The first of these campaigns under the sponsorship of Nathan Straus, owner of Macy's, stirred up other concerns. Among them was the alarming infant death rate, then higher than that in any other developed country in the world. A series of investigations launched by members of the New York Milk Committee came to the conclusion that improving health for mothers and babies meant beginning with pregnancy.

In 1918 the Maternity Center Association was founded by a coalition of professional and lay reformers. Francis Perkins from the Children's Bureau (and later Secretary of Labor in Franklin Roosevelt's cabinet) was appointed executive secretary. Neighborhood clinics were set up where mothers could receive prenatal care and learn through small classes and demonstrations how to care for themselves and their infants. At that time birth was not readily discussed, and being pregnant was considered somehow shameful, so women tended to keep out of sight once their bulging bellies were obvious. In a brief history of childbirth education prepared for the International Childbirth Education Association, Virginia Larsen and Margaret Gamper described MCA nurses canvassing door to door and hanging around tenement grocery stores hoping to snare pregnant women and persuade them to come to a clinic.

Many of the women would otherwise have received no care at all during pregnancy. The success of MCA efforts was almost immediately evident. A study by Metropolitan Life three years later showed that among women receiving prenatal care, 21.5 percent fewer died in childbirth, and they lost 29.2 percent fewer babies. A subsequent study by the same company in 1930 showed that the death rate for women in the Bellevue Yorkville area of New York City was 2.4 per thousand for those enrolled in MCA classes, against 6.2 for those who were not.[28]

In 1923 Hazel Corbin was appointed general director of the association, a post she retained for forty-two years. As innovative and resourceful as she was enduring, she initiated and oversaw many programs designed to answer the shifting needs of American mothers. One of these was the Lobenstine Midwifery Clinic, established in 1931 as a facility for teaching midwifery to public health nurses so that they could supervise the immigrant and rural midwives still practicing at the time. The clinic-school was a memorial to Dr. Lobenstine, member of the MCA medical board, who had envisioned it as one factor in a larger plan to bring trained midwives "under competent medical control."[29]

In spite of this implied assurance that the training would produce midwives willing to submit to medical authority, there was an outburst of opposition and protest resignations from the MCA medical board whose members apparently feared that nurse midwives would threaten their control of obstetrics. It was many years (1971) before nurse midwives achieved even grudging recognition from the medical establishment, but the MCA and its Lobenstine Clinic persisted. Eventually the school became a resource center for training programs elsewhere, serving communities that Mary Breckenridge would have called the surviving American frontier. That usually meant areas where the poor of various minorities scrabbled for a living and where midwives were tolerated because they offered no competition to fee-for-service physicians. Among the institutions aided by the MCA were the Catholic Maternity Institute in Santa Fe, New Mexico, and the School for Midwives in Tuskegee, Alabama. A few Lobenstine graduates practiced midwifery in rural areas, but because nurse midwives had such a long battle for the right to practice, most became supervisors, teachers and consultants to governments here and abroad.

In the early 1970s, the MCA once again broke new ground in establishing a free-standing birth center in the basement of their headquarters on New York City's upper West Side. Although approval had been sought and received from various public health agencies for the project, there was another storm of opposition from the medical board, and a third of the members resigned in protest. (Chapter Five contains a more complete story of the MCA birth center and nurse midwives.)

MCA is noted for several other significant contributions to childbirth reform and education. In 1939, under its sponsorship, a prize was offered for the best drawings of fetal growth and development. Winning entries were to be exhibited at the World's Fair in New York City. A progressive and talented physician-artist, Robert L. Dickinson, won the award. He and sculptor Abram Belski produced life-size models of the fetus in progressive stages of labor based on Dickinson's drawings. Dickinson hand-carried these models to the Fair, traveling by train. Curious about the figures shrouded in newspaper wrappings, passengers inquired, and Dickinson seized the opportunity to give anatomy lessons on the spot. In an era when the vagina was termed the "birth passage" to erase its sexual connotation, and pregnancy was mentioned only in whispers, there was fierce opposition to displaying the life-size models in public. Maternity Center nurses had to whip up support from physicians in order to justify their exhibit. Even then, they had to remain constantly on call at the display to give medical aid to those who grew faint from the sight of a plaster baby in a plaster womb. Later photographs of the models were made into a series of charts called *The Birth Atlas* which has become the standard depiction of life before birth. After forty years, it continues to be used as a major visual aid in childbirth education in many countries of the world.

## Grantly Dick-Read: Prophet of Reclaiming Birth

The Maternity Center was also responsible for bringing the natural childbirth advocate Grantly Dick-Read to America for lectures in 1947. Read, known primarily in the U.S. as the author of *Childbirth Without Fear*, based his work on the theory that fear produces tension, and tension produces pain. Although the most prominent authority, he was not the first to describe this relationship. One predecessor, Mary Ries Melendy, a woman doctor educated at both regular and eclectic medical colleges in the Chicago area, wrote in *Sex-Life, Love, and Marriage* in 1913 that much of labor pain was caused by "tension, fear, lack of right knowledge, and inherited ignorance."[30] And there were other observers who suspected the same cause and effect but none who fashioned the theory into a philosophy of birth management and made its dissemination a life-work as Read did.

The sixth of seven children, he was brought up in an extremely pious upper middle-class English family who spent half of each year on a farm in East Anglia. His solitary habits in childhood and his fondness for observing the minutiae of nature on the rims of Norfolk marshes started him on the path to unorthodoxy. Later, several specific occurrences shaped his belief that the pains of labor were not of nature's making. The first took place during his internship in a London hospital when he attended a young woman in labor out on White Chapel Road. The woman lay on a makeshift bed in a wretched room where rain seeped through broken windows. During the final moments of a calm labor, she astonished the young intern by refusing his offer of a chloroform mask. Later she said, as if apologizing for having asserted herself, that the birth hadn't hurt, adding in what became Read's motto, "It wasn't meant to, was it?"[31]

Some years later, as an army surgeon during World War I, Read came across a Flemish woman giving birth alone in a field. She, too, refused his offer of aid, so he sat down and smoked a pipe while the woman, half-lying, half-sitting, brought forth her baby. When the cord blanched, she severed it neatly with her fingers, wrapped the child in a cloth, and waited for the placenta which emerged shortly with no bleeding that Read could see. He hastened away to get help in transporting the woman, and failing, returned to the countryside where he met her calmly walking along the road with her newborn in her arms.

His curiosity aroused by these two apparently painless births, Read made further observations as a resident senior obstetrician in London after the War. He developed the concept of a cycle of fear during labor leading to tension and tension to pain, in turn producing more fear. In light of current theories on the close connection between body and mind, few would question such a formula; in the thirties, it constituted an assault on accepted medical thought. Advised not to publish his notes on the dozens of labors that supported his theory, Read stubbornly continued to submit the manuscript to one publisher after another. Finally one agreed to print the book if the author paid for part of the expense. At the time, Read, specializing in obstetrics, was in clinic practice with three other physicians. As soon as his book gained publicity, his partners dissolved the arrangement and brought charges of unprofessional conduct against him. After a year of wrangling, the charges were eventually settled in Read's favor, but during that time he had been barred from practice.

Afterwards, reviled, accused of promoting cruelty to women, of using secret, mystical hypnosis, he could hardly find any patients at all. He was refused academic posts for which he was qualified and was blocked from hospitals where he needed to test his theory further. Under the stress, the pain and crippling of wounds he had suffered at Gallipoli during the War flared again so he could barely walk. In spite of this, he continued to fight for his ideas. With the support and encouragement of a secretary who later became his second wife, Jessica Read, he felt he'd found his mission in life. He believed that he was "right" in the same way that other medical pioneers had been right and been persecuted for it—Semmelweis, Lister, Pasteur.

A hundred years earlier, another British doctor had been harassed for daring to tamper with childbirth practices. That was James Simpson of Edinburgh who on January 19, 1847, poured a half teaspoonful of chloroform on a handkerchief and held it over the nose of a woman in labor, thus setting off a fierce controversy. Simpson was attacked for daring to circumvent the Biblical condemnation of women to childbed agony, whereas a century later Read was attacked just as bitterly for proposing that instruction in relaxation might enable women to endure labor without painkillers. In the nineteenth century argument which raged briefly between clergymen and doctors, doctors appeared as the champions of womankind, while religious leaders declared that birth pain was necessary to produce motherly love. The religious case was weakened in 1853 when Queen Victoria asked for chloroform for the birth of her seventh child, Prince Leopold (whose subsequent sickliness was sometimes blamed on the drug). However, in 1949 Princess Elizabeth's reported interest in natural ·birth for her first child did not prove so helpful to Read. Sir William Gilliat, president of the Royal College of Obstetricians and Gynecologists (and Elizabeth's personal obstetrician), hinted broadly that if Read wanted a place to test his theories he ought to find another country in which to work.[32]

In America the response from physicians was equally unreceptive.

In the first article of the *Ladies' Home Journal* series previously cited, De Kruif acknowledged Read's pioneering work in returning childbirth to a more natural course. However, he, like his mentor DeLee, clearly considered the theory irrelevant to the task at hand which was to lower the maternal death rate and upgrade the obstetric specialty. Having babies easily and without drugs, according to De Kruif, might be possible for "your savage woman," who, having grown up with hardship and pain in her daily life, was prepared to labor hard to produce her baby. "But for your civilized woman the travail of the coming of her first baby is usually the first fundamental event in life she can't put off onto others, can't possibly run away from."[33] And this woman, according to De Kruif and DeLee and countless others, could not readily be trained back to the "fearless naturalness of savages." First of all, obstetricians would have to be educated in the new science so that they could then train the women, who, of course, could not learn on their own. And that process would take, according to DeLee, several thousand generations.[34]

In the thirties and forties, most of the women who were aware of the controversy would have agreed with DeLee. Generally, they were not anxious to return to what their grandmothers had suffered, as demonstrated by indignant letters to *The Times* following Gertrude Neilson's speech in 1936. Furthermore, they felt that undrugged childbirth was crude and unscientific, and as modern women they wanted no part of it. Nor would they accept the dictum that their greatest ecstasy and triumph in life would come from being awake to hear their infant's first cry, as Read insisted.

Nevertheless, his theories survived, largely because of concern over drugs which prompted some women and a few doctors to look for other solutions to labor pain. At that time, a variety of drugs in various combinations were being used in labor and delivery rooms, a situation which struck one observer as highly suspicious. According to this doctor, a visitor from Sweden, a scheme which had been worked out following the best medical standards ought not to allow twenty ways of getting the same result. In an article containing the Swedish doctor's views, the journalist describes one of the recipes for painless birth used in 1940:

(The physician would) smother the grinding pains of the first stage with a little scopolamine and barbiturate, going on with an enema of alcohol, ether and oil, ending with final-moment ether, and episiotomy, probably using forceps. To handle all that with proper care takes so large a staff of doctors and nurses that only crack and lavishly staffed hospitals can do the job.[35]

Few hospitals could offer such a staff or equipment, yet women continued to demand obliteration from pain, and the journalist, commenting on that reality, concluded that the only hope was that American women would adopt a more constructive attitude toward childbirth in the future. Read had already provided a philosophical base for new attitudes and some techniques for achieving them; however, it was nearly a decade before his theories were widely circulated in this country.

In 1946, *Colliers*, a popular weekly magazine, published an article about a doctor named Blackwell Sawyer who had been using Read methods in rural New Jersey since 1943. He had impulsively offered what he'd learned from Read's book to a woman in the throes of a painful labor. Initial success led him further, and by 1946 he had taught some one hundred sixty-eight women how to minimize pain. In the magazine article, titled "Motherhood without Misery," the author praised what he called the Read-Sawyer method, while noting a drawback in the need for a good deal of instruction from the attending doctor. Perhaps, he wrote, public health nurses could be trained to teach women how to control fear.[36]

## Margaret Gamper: Pioneer Childbirth Educator

In Chicago, a registered nurse who had in March 1946, given birth using what she herself had gleaned from reading Read's first book, was encouraged in a new and daring project by the *Colliers* article. Using it to bolster her argument, she persuaded her employer, an obstetrician-gynecologist, to let her teach the methods to his pregnant patients. Reluctantly he agreed, and Margaret Gamper, trained in the twenties to fill the subservient and submissive role of nurse, embarked on a new career which was to lead her to greater and greater independence and eventually to her own business as a childbirth educator.

In 1979, after more than thirty years in the field, Margaret talked with some other childbirth educators about her history. To their surprise, she said she had entered the field by accident; she had really wanted to work with menopausal women. However, for almost as long as she could remember, and certainly since the day in 1918 when she saw her brother brought home for burial, she had wanted to be a nurse.

She was born Margaret Hilt, June 2, 1907, in Janesville, Wisconsin, the seventh in a family of nine. Margaret remembered her mother, a woman of imposing girth, as often seated in a large wicker rocking chair that was festooned with bags of her handiwork. The Hilt children, returning from school on Wisconsin winter afternoons, delighted in warming their hands under Ma's large arms and in begging for pennies from a small leather bag she kept suspended from a string around her neck.

Mr. Hilt ran his own successful business as a general contractor and stone mason in Janesville. When Margaret was five or six, he tried his hand at homesteading in Montana. The family went along, but Margaret stayed only a few months. Considered too sickly for ranch life, she was sent back to Janesville to live with a married sister, Nell. For the next five years, she saw little of her mother and came to think of herself as belonging in some special way to Nell.

When the United States entered World War I, the older boys were eager to join the fight. Mr. Hilt, unable to manage the ranch alone, gave it up, and the family returned to Janesville. Frank, the second son, was the first to go to war. A few months later the Hilts received word from an Army camp in Waco, Texas, that he was dead, a victim of the great influenza epidemic of 1918. His body, representing Janesville's first casualty of the War, was shipped back for a hero's burial. After a funeral at home, the flag-covered casket was borne to the cemetery in a glass-paneled hearse drawn by black horses. Margaret watched the ceremonies for her brother with a mixture of grief and awe, and vowed she would serve her country as he had done. She couldn't fight, but she could be a nurse and tend the wounded.

Life was fairly easygoing in Janesville in the prosperous years following the War, and Margaret grew up accepting some things as quite ordinary. Women casually opened their dresses to breastfeed without shocking anyone, and sometimes Margaret would find a pregnant woman in the family kitchen, her dress up around her neck while Mrs. Hilt, who was famous for predicting a baby's sex before birth, examined the swollen belly for clues. She never explained to her daughters how the woman had gotten into that condition because any child with eyes in her head could deduce that by watching dogs in the street.

Still, certain events such as menstruation had to be prepared for. After bringing home a supply of huck towels, Mrs. Hilt told fourteen-year-old Margaret how they were to be placed between the legs and pinned to a rag belt. The soiled towels had to be washed privately and dried out of sight behind the barn where no one could see their blood stains bleaching in the sun. At such times Margaret, like the other girls, must wear a rubber apron tied the wrong way around under her clothing to keep anything from seeping through. Margaret, mystified by all the secrecy and precaution, had to wait another two years before she needed her huck towels.

An inventive and romantic child, her favorite occupation was reading love stories in the pulp magazines she pilfered from her mother and read on the sly, stories in which things always turned out happily. In real life that wasn't so. When Nell became bedfast with chronic nephritis, Margaret was chosen to stay home from school to nurse her and care for her little boy, and she stayed home again to take care of her mother, ill with diphtheria. "My family," she said later, "made a nurse of me long before I entered training." Her responsibilities increased as Nell's health worsened, and Margaret fell further behind in school. When she was sixteen, the sister who had been mother to her died.

Early in 1927, Margaret finally completed requirements for a high school diploma. Determined to keep the promise she had made at Frank's death, she saved money for living expenses during nurses training by doing piecework in Janesville industries. In one factory she sewed lace on brassieres for wages of thirty-five cents a dozen, and in another she made shades for Chevrolet automobile windows.

When the youngest Hilt child, Mary, died of appendicitis at the age of twelve, Mrs. Hilt decided she was not going to lose any more children if she could help it. Margaret, who had been accepted as a probationer at a hospital in Detroit, received a letter shortly thereafter canceling the acceptance. Bitterly disappointed by the rejection, Margaret might not have known the reason had she not come quietly into the house one day and overheard her mother talking to a friend. Mrs. Hilt confided she had written the hospital saying she'd lost two daughters and didn't want to lose another; would they please help by refusing Margaret's application?

In a fury, Margaret rushed to the home of an older brother and his German wife. The young woman, who had worked with Margaret at Chevrolet, knew her mother-in-law despised her for being German. In retaliation she helped Margaret run away to become a student nurse in Chicago. The elder Hilts knew nothing of their daughter's whereabouts until later in the year when Margaret was forced to ask their permission for surgery after an appendicitis attack. Mr. Hilt came to Chicago to sign the necessary papers, and while he never actually forgave her for running away, he said she was the only child in the family who had inherited his gumption. With her father's unspoken blessing, Margaret was on her own.

In the twenties, student nurses endured lives of backbreaking labor, governed by a network of strict rules that did not protect them from harassment. In spite of a bright ready smile, Margaret was considered a "frozen chicken" among the interns for whom all student nurses were fair game. On one occasion an intern chased her into the diet kitchen where Margaret leaped up on a steam table. When the intern attempted to drag her down, she swung out on an exposed pipe and kicked the hapless man so forcibly in his "parts" that he had to be carried away by fellow interns while Margaret watched in shock and fear of punishment.

During training, Margaret and other students had followed their director from Washington Park to Illinois Masonic Hospital, and there in March 1931, Margaret completed training and passed the state examination. She was granted an R.N. in July of that year. The country was sliding deeper into the Depression, and jobs were scarce. After weeks of searching, Margaret found work as a private duty nurse with no pay but bed and board—bed being a cot kept under the patient's bed during the day. Eventually, she was hired to work in admitting and receiving at Cook County Hospital where the poor of the populous county came for medical attention, often in emergency. A doctor noticed the young nurse's skill in patching people up, and advised her to take a post-graduate course in surgical techniques. She finished the six-month course and, discovering she had a talent for surgery, went on to advanced training in operating room supervision.

While still a student, Margaret met Hugo Gamper, a young man who worked for the Illinois Central Railway. In spite of parental opposition on both sides, the couple eloped in 1935 and settled down to married life in a Chicago suburb. While she was hoping for her first baby, Margaret cast about for projects to keep her busy. This was the beginning of years of longing for pregnancy, of weeping each month when it did not occur, but she continued to work. In 1938, Harold W. Miller, an obstetrician-gynecologist, asked her to serve as his assistant, not only in surgery but by making rounds of his hospital patients and visiting those confined at home. Proving herself capable of even more responsibility, Mrs. Gamper was soon changing dressings, taking out stitches, and gathering histories and notes on patients in three hospitals. In addition, she traveled around Chicago by streetcar visiting Miller's homebound patients, those who were threatened with miscarriage, and others who were simply too depressed and immobilized by menopause to go outside.

Most of the older women were disheveled and apologetic, no longer hopeful enough to comb their hair in honor of Mrs. Gamper's visit. She began to take more time with the hormone injections, pausing to chat with the women, telling them about herself and inviting them to respond. "I dressed in fashionable suits, not nurse uniforms because that made me appear more like a friend. I'd get them (the older women) to fix themselves up and take renewed interest in the world."

Seeing that a back rub, a facial, and help with makeup worked wonders for the women's self-esteem, Margaret embarked on a series of evening classes leading to a diploma from the American School of Beauty Culture. Using what she learned as she went along, she eventually took the state board examination. Returning to night school again, she completed a course in the Swedish College of Massage and Physical Therapy.

Meanwhile, Hugo was being promoted to better positions with the railway, but the Gampers' climb up the economic ladder did not make up for the grief of childlessness and attempts to cure it. Margaret consulted specialists, followed courses of hormone therapy and endured tubal insufflations. Finally, in the summer of 1941, she found herself pregnant and happily worked through the fall and into winter. On what was to be her last day of work in January 1942, a truck skidded on the icy pavement and struck her car. Shaken but seemingly uninjured, she went home. That evening she began to bleed, and for the next two weeks lay in an elevated bed in the hospital, trying unsuccessfully to hang on to the baby. She lost her infant son in the sixth month of pregnancy.

The next few months were grim. Depressed and underweight, Margaret returned to work but refused to go on the obstetrical wards or see maternity patients until Dr. Miller insisted. Soon afterward, she was pushing a surgical cart with its dressings and antiseptics down an incline into the maternity ward when it tipped over, spilling a flood of merthiolate. The widening pool of red reminded Margaret of the loss of her child, and she ran from the ward crying uncontrollably. After taking her home, Miller persuaded her to see another physician, an eminent gynecologist sympathetic to women. In his office she sobbed out the story of her years of barrenness, the dead baby, and the longing that consumed all her thoughts and energies. The doctor advised her to let go her urgency for a baby and return to her profession. Eased by his understanding, she made an effort to recover her health and went back to work.

Three years later Margaret became pregnant in her thirty-ninth year and this time carried the baby to term. One day she made a house call on a pneumonia patient who also happened to be pregnant. Margaret found the woman sitting up in bed reading Read's *Childbirth Without Fear* and asked if they could study together. Later she watched the woman go through a short easy labor and give birth without interference. The woman's conviction that having a baby was a natural and even beautiful event seemed to make labor easier.

A few weeks later, Margaret happened on another woman in labor who was doing breathing exercises. "Are you trying to have a natural birth?" Margaret asked. The woman replied briskly that she wasn't *trying*—she was, in fact, doing so. Confident that the woman would soon be begging for pain-killers, her obstetrician and other staff members watched in astonishment as she proceeded through a spontaneous delivery without their help.

On March 27, 1946, bolstered by Read's book and those few observations, Margaret also went through labor without drugs or interference and gave birth to a daughter who became known in the years following by Margaret's own phrase: "The child who made love visible." Taking Mary Jane with her so she could breastfeed, Margaret soon was back making house calls. Late in the year she came across the *Colliers* article on Sawyer and his successful use of Read methods. Struck by the ignorance and fear she saw daily among women in childbirth and convinced that Read relaxation would work for them, too, Margaret organized her first class of eight women, all Dr. Miller's patients.

Dr. Miller remained skeptical, even appalled as his enthusiastic assistant made plans to show a 1930 birth film to a mixed audience of expectant mothers and fathers. What, he wanted to know, would be Mr. White's response if he had to sit beside Mrs. Green while they were both compelled to look at Mrs. Brown's upturned and naked bottom? Margaret didn't know what the response would be, but she was willing to risk it. Unconvinced, Dr. Miller elected to stay outside, pacing nervously through the hall. To her surprise and certainly his, at that first showing the men in the audience seemed more appreciative and inclined to comment than the women.

Read's visit to the United States the following year, including an appearance in Chicago, spurred more public interest, and attendance at Margaret's classes increased. By 1949, she and her successful method were becoming known well enough to warrant feature articles in Chicago newspapers.[37] That same year she wrote and produced a film on her relaxation method—the first of five Gamper films.

When Mary Jane outgrew her car seat and could no longer be easily carried about from house calls to hospitals, the Gampers hired an older woman to cook and clean and play with the little girl. Remaining for fourteen years, the housekeeper became a member of the family, an adopted grandmother from whom Margaret learned skills she would use and teach years later. She concentrated all her efforts on her work as a childbirth educator and in 1955 broke with Miller, an unprecedented move in an era when nurses seldom set up an independent practice. Her enterprise was first called Cradleland and later the Midwest Parentcraft Center. When it became known that 95 percent of the women in Gamper classes delivered without medication, some doctors began to recommend her to their patients. Others refused to have anything to do with her. One obstetrician reported her to the local medical society as a hypnotist, but later sent an asthmatic patient to her for instruction in labor breathing.

Although well-schooled in traditional deference to physicians, Margaret launched an attempt to change birth practices in an area still heavily under the influence of Dr. DeLee and his conviction that pregnancy and labor were diseased conditions. By the late forties, the time allotted to second-stage labor had been so curtailed through the use of episiotomy and forceps that few women were given more than thirty minutes in the delivery room. In theory, this was to save the infant from a cruel battering against its mother's perineum; in practice, it also made for more efficient use of hospital facilities. Aware that her advocacy of a more natural course ran counter to the convenience of the institutions, Margaret moved slowly, convinced she could persuade by good-humored persistence.

As she directed Cradleland, she began to discover her own independent voice and style. Putting together a package of skills she derived from Read, her training in Swedish massage and physical therapy, and infused with a view of nursing in its best sense as the laying on of hands, Margaret wrote and published her first book, *Relax, Here's Your Baby*, in 1951. For many years it remained the only book on childbirth education by an American nurse, and it bravely discussed and depicted birth from a woman's point of view during a time when anything frank about the female body was considered poor taste. She used the book almost solely as a text for her own classes and, as with the films, never attempted national distribution. In any event, her work was either unknown or unacknowledged by members of the nursing profession who tended to overlook accomplishments not sponsored by the medical profession. However, she was noticed in other circles. When the International Childbirth Education Association came into being in 1960, Margaret was one of the first members, and as she had been conducting classes and training sessions for more than a decade, was asked to be on the board of consultants.

While Margaret was known as a Read follower, she sometimes did not receive credit for other innovative work. For a time she was intrigued by "Birtheeze," a plastic suit that removed pressure from the uterus with consequent reduction of pain and theoretically increased oxygen supply to the fetus. Although the Birtheeze was never widely used in America, its principles were incorporated in some types of labor breathing. Gamper added them in her classes "quite by accident," and in *Preparation for the Heir-minded* written in 1971, described the technique:

> The uterus is practically ellipoid (oval) in shape, with the upper segment tilted backward from the lower segment. During a contraction, the uterus tends to become spherical (round) and rises forward. A tense abdominal wall resists these changes causing the contracting uterus to expend a good portion of its energy overcoming this resistance. Decompression produces relaxation by mechanical means and is not affected by the mother's emotions. . . . Quite by accident before I ever heard of the birth suit (1949), I discovered how to hold the abdominal wall up. . . . While assisting one of my students . . . I slid my hands underneath her tired back to rub. . . . As I withdrew my hands . . . I lifted upward toward the ceiling. My patient was delighted. . . . I had mighty tired hands and arms for the next couple of years.[38]

Margaret eventually taught fathers how to lift their wives' abdomens and later devised "shelf and bulge" techniques where women could lift their own abdomens during a contraction. Although intrigued by the Birtheeze, she returned to the belief that it was best to cope with labor by simple means without external devices to distract the women.

*Preparation* reflects Margaret's respect for medical authority, but at the same time she urged her readers to action and independence. "Do not let anyone sway or deter you from your important goal unless there is sound medical reason for intervention. . . . The use of drugs during labor is unfair to the mother and her baby. . . . "[39] She included the story of a father denied access to the delivery room unless he submitted to a battery of costly tests, including stool examination, throat culture, and X-rays. He took all the tests required and then demanded that everyone else who was to be in the delivery room do likewise—doctors, nurses, aides, and orderlies—with the results sent to his attorney. Needless to say, that father was allowed to witness the birth of his child without any further hindrance. Others, the author implied, could do the same.

Over the years, Margaret collected an impressive library of old and rare books on obstetrics, including an eighteenth-century English edition of Aristotle's *Complete and Experienced Midwife* and an American manual, *The Practice of Midwifery*, published in 1833. From these books and her own observation and experience, she gained a long-range view of obstetrical care, of the ebb and flow of technology, and of the perennial argument that whatever the latest invention, it would produce better pregnancies and births. A footnote in a 1980 edition of her newsletter for present and former students comments on a discussion on Bendectin, a morning sickness drug that has been charged with causing birth defects. "It appears that the conservative treatments of the good old days for nausea and vomiting will return just as Mom's chicken soup and commonsense have for the ordinary cold."[40]

In the seventies, finding herself short of young mothers to act as volunteer staff for the Center, Margaret recruited grandmothers, some from monthly classes in the art of grandmothering which she had originated. A long-time widow, Margaret knew that life was hard for traditionally raised women who found themselves suddenly on their own. She taught these older women that young mothers need their help and encouragement and that they must develop the confidence and knowledge to offer aid.

In 1979, as trim and fashionably dressed as always, Margaret appeared at a regional ICEA conference to speak on the subject of grandmothering. First she asked each grandmother in the audience to describe her own experience in giving birth. Most told the same story of being drugged during labor and left alone in a hospital room to endure a confusing, painful, and frightening event. Then tending the projector, Margaret showed the slow-paced black and white film she had made in 1946 when she herself was a new mother. Efficient in white scrub dress, the younger Margaret assists a woman giving birth, while the present Margaret described how all traces of urine had been removed from the patient's bladder by catheter, how she was shaved clean, a practice deemed necessary to get rid of pubic lice, and how her bottom was painted scarlet with antiseptics to kill germs and prevent infection. On a bedside table, a padded tongue depressor is evident for use if the woman convulsed during labor, a reminder of the days when eclampsia was common.

The white-haired Margaret continued to narrate, explaining how warm wet compresses were placed against the woman's perineum to aid in stretching it out for the birth of the baby, since the attending doctor, Margaret's employer, did not make routine episiotomies. In the film, Margaret supports the woman's legs so she can push. The woman is fully conscious and smiling, almost passive in Margaret's arms. There seems to be very little panting and no explosive breaths. Although it was generally routine in the forties to extract babies with forceps, in this case the physician does not use instruments at all. Margaret drew attention to the fact that there was a minor loss of blood during the birth, as compared with bleeding in an anesthetized woman. The labor continues on film, young Margaret working almost as hard as the mother, lifting her with each contraction and encouraging her. Margaret described the woman as giving birth with "nature telling her the way, guided along the definite patterns established by a labor where there is no intervention, doing the simple breathing as it fits her needs."

When the film finished, the surreal effect of watching an older woman project her thirty years' younger self on the screen vanished, leaving a sharpened awareness of Margaret Gamper's impressive contribution to the childbirth education movement during those same decades. Before the childbirth reform movement gained momentum in the sixties, she stood alone in the unique position of a nurse turned childbirth educator. In addition to the classes in the Gamper method, the books, films, and seminars, she trained dozens of nurses to become childbirth teachers on their own and encouraged many people, including Dr. Robert Bradley of Denver, along the way. In her low key fashion she has continued to nudge parents into taking more initiative in seeking the kind of childbirth care they would like to have. Through all this she has maintained the deep trust in the wholeness of the body and the flowing processes by which it gives birth that is the hallmark of the true Read teacher.

# TWO

# The Stirrings of Protest
# 1950-1970

The years following World War II have been described as a time of reaction and return to traditional values in American homes— the era of privatization, Betty Friedan called it.[1] During the War, women had cut their hair, shortened their skirts, and gone out to replace men in factories and fields and offices. Now they put on tight-waisted long-skirted dresses in styles reminiscent of the nineteenth century and came back home to cook, clean house, and most of all to have babies. Birth almost always took place in hospitals under the supervision of physicians. The advice and experiences of the older generation had long since been discarded as out-of-date and irrelevant, as though the biological process itself had been revised. In all areas, American women listened to instructions from an army of experts: psychologists, sociologists, anthropologists, child behavior experts, sex experts, and, of course, medical doctors. In childbearing, the obstetrician was considered an unquestioned authority on all matters, from diet and weight gain through the psychological and emotional needs during pregnancy and labor, including what most women assumed was an accurate assessment of what having a baby felt like at any given moment.

The battle during the twenties and thirties for painless birth through drugs appeared to be won so completely that women lost all memory of having been protagonists against the medical men, of ever having insisted on some influence in the conduct of their labors. The need for submission to medical control was seldom challenged.

In the *Ladies' Home Journal*, a popular feature was titled, "Tell Me, Doctor." In each issue the author, Henry B. Safford, discussed a feminine medical problem with an anonymous patient. In a series on birth, he responded to the woman's query about whether her doctor would stay with her during labor:

> "If he's a busy man he may have other patients to serve at the same time. However, you need have little fear that he'll neglect you. It won't help much to have him sit by the bedside and hold your hand throughout labor—in fact, such a procedure would be good neither for you nor for him. It is far better that he come in with a fresh point of view at the time when he is needed. His judgement will as a rule be better than if he had been watching you helplessly for hours. . . . "
> "Can I have my family with me?"
> "Certainly not. Your husband might be permitted to see you for a short interval from time to time, but as to anyone else—not if I can help it. One of the very good reasons for being in a hospital is to get away from well-meaning but uninformed advisors."
> "That sounds sort of cruel."
> "It's not. It's kind. Well, now, we've got through the first stage . . . "[2]

With this brisk dismissal of the woman's anxiety about being left alone and a reiteration of DeLee's 1916 injunction: "No babbling relatives or friends should be allowed in the room,"[3] the Tell-Me-Doctor went on to describe the rest of the process from his point of view:

> "Let's say that we have reached the point where the patient feels great pressure in the region of the outlet . . . Now is the time when she must be taken to the delivery room and made ready for the actual birth event. There she is placed upon a specially devised table equipped with stirrups, which sustain her legs with knees flexed in an appropriate position for delivery. Her hands are also effectively restrained. (Here the woman interrupts to protest the thought of being bound hand and foot.) It amounts to that, and the reason is that you will shortly be going to sleep and it is desired to restrain whatever involuntary movements you might make so that the sterility setup may not be broken. . . . Now the delivery is ready to take place and this will be managed slowly and carefully by your doctor, while you are sound asleep. . . . In all probability you will know nothing or feel nothing until you suddenly awake and hear, coming from what will probably seem a great distance, a lusty little 'Wa-a-ah!' . . . "[4]

Childbirth in which the woman was efficiently removed as an intelligent being was most common during this period and was most often described by medical personnel since they were the only conscious observers. However, we have the view of another sort of observer in the recollection of Lester Hazell who wangled her way into the delivery room of Georgetown University Hospital where she was working as a technician in the early fifties. The birthing woman, expecting her sixth child, had told Lester earlier that all the other births were perfect because she had known nothing until some hours afterward when her new baby, clean and snugly wrapped, was brought to her. By the time Lester entered the delivery room, the woman was already unconscious, legs raised and propped apart in stirrups, and a spotlight shining on the one undraped portion of her body, the bloody gap at her groin. Doctors and nurses working over her were as remote from the event as mechanics tinkering with an automobile engine. They talked of sports and a party while the woman snored on. The obstetrician inserted a shiny metal spoon in the woman's vagina, and then another, and clamping them together, tugged with great effort until he pulled out a limp, blue infant. The baby did not cry until slapped smartly on the behind. Then it stiffened and looked about itself with interest. Lester, wonder-struck at the sight of a new life, felt that of all those in the gleaming and sterile chamber, only she and the baby knew what had just happened. The other participants chattered on behind their masks as unaware of the moment as the drugged and dreaming mother.[5]

There were other modes of giving birth in American hospitals but aside from accidents, they were generally available only to a few who happened on an experimental project in Read theories. The best known of these took place at Grace-New Haven Hospital in a collaboration between Yale Medical Center and the Maternity Center Association, under the direction of Herbert Thoms, head of ob-gyn at Yale. Every other patient at the clinic was assigned to a program involving classes for both parents, tours of the facilities and preparation for a natural, that is, physiological birth. Several women whose names have slipped out of sight contributed significantly to the Yale project. Physiotherapist Helen Heardman and her book *A Way to Natural Childbirth* provided basic material for prenatal classes. When on tour of the United States with Read in 1947, she herself instructed obstetric nurses in breathing and relaxation techniques. Heardman was "our first instructors' instructor" according to Mary Lempke, a childbirth educator who was a student nurse at Yale that year. Certified nurse midwives from the Maternity Center and Dr. Edith Jackson designed the rooming-in project in which one nurse was responsible for the care and education of four mothers and their infants.[6] Thoms' beliefs, strongly influenced by Read, provided a philosophy for the whole program. He viewed birth as a natural phenomenon, one in which a woman's "whole being—her emotions as well as her body—is engaged in a wonderfully subtle, creative endeavor. She is in the midst of the greatest moments of her life."[7]

One woman who participated in the study during her first pregnancy in 1950 recalled a somewhat different message. "Everything was oriented toward treating the whole birth experience as part of our normal lives." This was well before the advent of the Pill, when contraception as well as abortion was illegal in many states, and pregnancy, welcome or not, overtook most women in the first few years of marriage. This young mother saw the Preparation for Childbirth Program as a superb method of teaching women how to cope with that inevitable occurrence. Unlike a friend who described the moment of birth in Readian terms of ecstasy, she experienced prepared delivery as a short period of "intense, concentrated, hard work," that was considerably eased by the support of friendly and sensitive staff members. In fact, people were what she remembered most of all, not the exercise classes, beneficial as they were, nor the decor which in her view remained dully institutional, but the doctors, nurses, and aides who treated participants as "individual, equal, human beings who were momentarily in need of their services and advice."[8]

Thoms felt that this radical shift in attitude was possible for all hospitals with relatively small upheaval and might come about if doctors would only demand the change. But few doctors saw the necessity.

One of the rare exceptions was Robert Bradley in Denver, who used modified Read principles in his private practice with notable success, achieving a national reputation. Assisted by Rhondda Hartman, a Canadian nurse who developed a program of exercises for his classes (*Exercises for True Natural Childbirth*), Bradley started with the idea that drugs used during pregnancy and birth cause a form of internal pollution. "I felt not only that these drugs were temporarily harmful to newborn babies—which is obvious at just a cursory glance—but also that a subtle depletion of brain function persists through the lifetime of the individual." His solution was to train human mothers to have babies as other mammals did. "With proper preparation human 'animals' can enjoy spontaneous unmedicated births."[9]

This preparation was to a large extent supervised by the husband acting as coach throughout pregnancy and labor. The Bradley method came to be called "Husband Coached Childbirth" which was the name of his book as well. Later critics accused Bradley of promoting a superior male alliance between obstetrician and husband formed to keep the "little woman" in line and behaving properly for the health of her child. In spite of his stalwart opposition to standard obstetrical practices, contemporary reformers tend to judge him harshly for his patronizing attitude such as his advice to fathers: "Let's face a fact: they're (pregnant women) nuttier than a fruitcake . . . "[10]

In Seattle in the late forties, Virginia Larsen, a physician and mother who had been distressed by her own experiences in childbirth — at one point the ward nurse had chastised Dr. Larsen severely for daring to unwrap the blanket in order to inspect her own little son — headed a Family Life class at the local YWCA in hope of promoting a different sort of birth. Encouraged by the response, she later borrowed money for bus fare and came East to study natural birth at the Maternity Center in New York and at Grace-New Haven. Her Seattle students, often young couples producing the large families of the post-war baby boom, were so enthusiastic about Dr. Larsen's skill in making birth a pleasant experience that they formed a continuing group to work for reform that later became a prototype for a national organization.

## Elisabeth Bing and the Lamaze Solution

In New York City during this same period, a physiotherapist was establishing her own practice as a Read educator. European-born and trained, Elisabeth Bing was totally on her own when she began tramping from the office of one obstetrician to another, asking for referrals of pregnant patients. A few doctors agreed. More thought she was crazy, although probably harmless. She persisted in her aim, even when the lack of patients meant taking a job as an office nurse to tide her over the first sparse years. Difficult times and sudden change had been the pattern of much of her adult life, and by then she had learned not only how to survive but how to do so with a certain grace.

She was born in 1914 in Germany to parents who were members of the respected German-Jewish intelligentsia. Her father, George Koenigsberger, was an architect for the city of Berlin, and he and his wife and five children lived in Gruenau, one of its suburban communities. Elisabeth remembered an idyllic childhood on the banks of the river Dahme. The half-timbered house, with gables, dormers and leaded windows, sat in a green lawn surrounded by chestnut and elm trees. On the river bank where weeping willows trailed in the current, the family boats were moored. There was a flat-bottom Norwegian scow that the children might use whenever they pleased and a canoe and sailboat that required permission. Once there had been a motor yacht, but it had been lost while Herr Koenigsberger was using it to patrol the Vistula River in Poland during World War I.

The affectionate and lively parents were interested in their children's development and read to them constantly. The father required that each child keep a drawing notebook and produce evidence of continuing achievement in art and other skills. It was assumed that all the children, girls as well as boys, would be educated for a profession in the family tradition. (One uncle, Max Born, was Nobel laureate.) But they also were expected to train themselves physically. Summers were spent on the water, swimming and rowing; winters occupied by academic studies at the gymnasium were enlivened by athletic competition. Elisabeth, naturally able, won a bronze award for her performance on the parallel bars.

This idyllic life came to an end in 1931 when Herr Koenigsberger fell mortally ill. Elisabeth and her younger brother were sent away to protect them from witnessing their father's decline. After his death, she completed studies at the gymnasium and enrolled at the University of Berlin in 1933. Two days later she was abruptly dismissed, "sacked because I was a Jew." For the young woman whose sense of her family's origins was more of culture than religion, this event was a considerable shock. Restless, she longed to be away and on her own and so was sent to Derbyshire in England where a family friend could keep an eye on her. Elisabeth never returned home to live. Before the end of the decade, all the rest of her immediate family had followed her out of Germany to safety.

Emulating a favorite aunt who was a physiotherapist, Elisabeth decided to train for that profession, but there was little money for tuition now that her father was dead and life was increasingly difficult for the family in Germany. One physical therapy school offered tuition credit for students who were willing to spend their first year as probationary nurses, so Elisabeth, fresh from a sheltered life in Gruenau, went to work on hospital wards in the English Midlands.

"We were treated like dirt," she said afterward. "We lived in a dormitory and were paid one shilling a day for ten to twelve hours' work. It was terrible."

The break from a life in which she had been cherished to one in which she was ordered about and forced to do menial ward work, empty bedpans, change soiled bedding and scrub floors was deeply humiliating. Lonely and feeling deserted, she fell ill with a mastoid infection. In London for surgery, she discovered a Quaker fund for refugees which enabled her to enroll in a physiotherapy school associated with two London hospitals. There students learned to give treatments in outpatient clinics and on the wards, most often to people who were severely disabled by polio and stroke. After working with patients whose outlook was grim, it was a relief to come on the maternity wards where women lay abed for eleven days following childbirth. Forbidden to even sit up and dangle their feet for the first week, they sometimes developed "milk leg" or thrombophlebitis from the inactivity. In order to prevent such problems, the physical therapy students massaged the women and instructed them in exercises, including what are now called "Kegels"— pelvic floor exercises to strengthen and heal vaginal muscles. Such exercises were not generally seen as useful for postpartum women for another twenty years, but Elisabeth learned them in 1933. At that time she was no more than casually interested in birth. Permitted to watch a delivery, she decided that having a baby, at least in an English hospital, was a rough experience.

In 1937 she received her license as a physical therapist, obtained work with a woman doctor and later moved on, free-lancing among various hospitals as a substitute for therapists who were ill or on holiday. Independent and aloof, she resisted becoming a permanent member of any one group. She married and moved into a comfortable flat in north London on the road that rises to Hampstead Heath. The marriage ended in divorce two years later but left its legacy in the flat in Belsize Park which remained for twenty years a London base for Elisabeth, her family and friends.

This was at the outset of World War II. Elisabeth, with her

German accent, had difficulty finding work in the first rush of patriotism. For a period, she had to leave London for Blackpool on the northwest coast but eventually returned when public hysteria had subsided into the long struggle to survive the air war. Sharing the flat with cousins, she settled into a precarious life that afterward seemed richer than any before or since.

The flat itself became a symbol of the life she and her friends were leading. There they endured night air raids, preferring the familiar rooms to the caverns of the underground railway station shelters. There they pooled ration coupons for the luxury of one Sunday roast a month which many were invited to share. When the electricity failed, they all trouped across the road to a friend's kitchen and his gas cooker. When the gas failed, he came to their flat, often bearing a huge pot of soup. Everyone took a weekly turn patrolling the block as fire warden. Everyone shared the horror of seeing a house, whole the day before, a ruin of rubble and shattered walls from a night bombing. Everyone participated in the talk of books, art and theatre, and in conversations fueled by the possibility of tomorrow's never coming. Many love affairs flared into existence during those months, and former lovers as well as current ones were welcomed. The charlady, scandalized by her young employers' freedom, managed to serve them and their overnight guests tea in the morning, but still breathed a great sigh of gratification when a flat member became engaged. "At least," she said, "one of you is doing the right thing."

In the year following the War's end, Elisabeth met an attractive Dutchman while she was staying at a ski resort on the continent. Despite his ill health, they married after a brief courtship, and Elisabeth returned with him to Holland where she learned the language well enough to work as a translator and proofreader for *Excerpta Medica*. She enjoyed the lively and tolerant life of post-war Amsterdam but soon knew the marriage had been a mistake. A few months later, her husband, who was much more seriously ill than she had known, died suddenly while Elisabeth was on a weekend visit to London. Suffering over both the mistaken marriage and her absence when he died, Elisabeth gathered herself together once again and returned to London to take up private practice as a therapist.

A patient who worked with the birth control movement gave Elisabeth a book she thought might interest her: *Childbirth without Fear*. Intrigued by Read's ideas, Elisabeth wondered whether the exercises she had taught women as a student might not be helpful during labor as well as afterward. She wrote to Read describing her training and interest and asked to meet him. He replied that she ought rather to see Helen Heardman, a physical therapist who was using his methods in hospitals in northern England. For various reasons, Elisabeth didn't make the journey, but her enthusiasm increased and she read every book on pregnancy she could find, although she didn't put her new expertise to use until she came to the United States on a visit in 1949.

Staying with a sister who had married and was living in a small university town in Illinois, Elisabeth worked as a therapist in a school for handicapped children. At a party she met a local obstetrician who was also interested in Read's theories. Elisabeth asked if he would send her some women to train for labor. He responded by sending all his pregnant patients and permitted Elisabeth to coach them through labor at the local hospital. Both were excited over the good results of her work. "It was great fun," Elisabeth said. But still, restless and feeling hemmed in by life in a small town, she decided to return to London. In what was meant only as a stopover in New York, she met Fred Bing, like herself a refugee from Germany. Their friendship grew and Elisabeth stayed on. After a year they married and settled into an apartment on Manhattan's West Side where they have remained for over thirty years. Life with Fred, who worked as a freight forwarder in overseas shipping, provided the first real security Elisabeth had known since her childhood in Gruenau. She wrote of this third marriage: "(it) meant a real settling down, almost like coming home. I had a real bedroom to sleep in for the first time in my adult life. No more sleeping on the living room couch. This felt like wonderful security."[11]

Now she began in earnest to establish herself as a Read childbirth educator. Popping up in one obstetrician's office after another, she became known in the city. When Alan Guttmacher, chief of obstetrics at Mt. Sinai Hospital, decided to establish prenatal classes, he hired her to head the program. Guttmacher, a nationally-known authority on pregnancy and an advocate of family planning, had emerged as a hero to the birth control movement after he invited the police to come and arrest him for dispensing illegal diaphragms in his clinic. He was not particularly interested in unmedicated births, only curious and tolerant enough to give Elisabeth a more or less free hand with her theories. The position offered immediate status and credibility, but she was not a registered nurse, and other women on the staff resented her, especially as Guttmacher gave her permission to stay with women throughout labor. Elisabeth, with her crazy foreign notions about easing pain through relaxation, was a natural target for resentment. She tried to keep out of the nurses' way and suppress an instinctively indignant response to the harassment. By that time she had learned that silence would better serve her cause.

"There was an obstetrics nurse, a supervisor whom everyone called a 'rough diamond.' We could hear her yelling three floors away. She was big and frightening and she called my work utter nonsense. I knew I was making progress when I heard her tell one of my students, 'Breathe, dammit, breathe. I wouldn't do it, but you are one of Mrs. Bing's patients, and you must. Breathe!' "

Working with Guttmacher took some forebearance, too. Despite his interest in her aims, he was arrogant and insensitive at times. Six foot four, he would stride swiftly along the corridors of Mt. Sinai while Elisabeth, more than a foot shorter, had to trot to keep up with him. And when she came to his office to confer, he might keep her cooling her heels while he finished the work at hand. Once so readily humiliated, Elisabeth had learned a confidence that enabled her to wait with some serenity.

Happily and securely married after all the years of upheaval, she and Fred, like the Gampers, longed for a child. After several early miscarriages and subsequent examinations for infertility, she inquired about adoption and was told that she and her husband, in their late thirties, were probably too old. While she lay at home in bed after a third miscarriage, she received word from London that her mother had died. This fresh grief combined with the other loss led her to ask her doctor if, for once, he could make a home visit. No, was the response. He was too busy. Elisabeth vowed to find someone who would take more interest.

The new doctor, also of German background and interested in natural birth, recommended a dilation and currement; when that was done, he pronounced Elisabeth quite healthy and fit to conceive and bear a child. Shortly afterward, whether from his reassurance or coincidence, she became pregnant and this time hung on as she "tiptoed through the first three months." Once the danger period passed, she and Fred entered a marvelous time of waiting for their baby. Never had New York seemed so inviting a city, so colorful and filled with promise.

When the time approached for delivery, Elisabeth, an expert

in preparation for others, discovered few resources for herself. This was 1955 when laboring women were still isolated and forbidden the support of a husband or anyone else in most hospitals. Remembering the many times nurses at Mt. Sinai had openly resented her privileges, she feared being at their mercy if she delivered there. She entered another hospital where no one knew her and where she was truly alone, with no other company than a vision of how an ideal labor ought to go. As an older first-time mother, or elderly primipara in medical jargon, she had expected a long, perhaps hard, labor, but she was physically fit and thought she could manage. Instead she went swiftly into a rough fast labor. Soon after admission, she found herself perched on a bedpan in a hot, damp communal bathroom while strangers walked in and out to use the toilets. She tried to control the forces at work in her body, but the ferocity of contractions and the sensations of the child turning and descending so quickly confused her. When the staff discovered that this patient, who had not screamed or otherwise indicated any such rapid progress, had dilated from two to ten centimeters in less than an hour, they hustled her off the bedpan, onto a gurney and into the delivery room.

On the delivery table, she was ordered to push and did so, but then abruptly her labor came to a stop, as sometimes happens when the mother is upset. Frantic that the baby might be damaged by delay, she asked over and over, "How is he? How is he?" No one answered, and finally the doctor, irritated by her questions, ordered her put out completely although she already had a spinal block. So the baby was delivered with forceps, and Elisabeth Bing missed the moment of birth that she had prepared for so well.

Recovery from a spinal required lying flat for twenty-four hours to avoid headaches caused by an imbalance in the spinal fluid. In Elisabeth's case, someone made a mistake, and she was told to get up as soon as she waked. The excruciating headache which resulted lasted eleven days, the same period of time English women had been kept in bed after childbirth. If she remembered that while she lay stone still avoiding the slightest movement, even blinking, because of the pain, Elisabeth reminded herself to be grateful that her child was, after all, healthy and alert after his disconcerting entry into the world. Despite the pain, she rolled to her side every four hours and nursed him, able at least to fulfill joyfully that part of her vision.

## The Fight Over Natural Childbirth

While Elisabeth Bing was developing and refining her work in teaching women how to prepare for labor, the controversy over the validity of Read's theories increased. Doctors, seeing natural childbirth as a threat to their control, attacked the motives and sanity of women who wanted to use the new techniques. As early as 1953, a group of Baltimore obstetricians wrote an article originally published in a medical journal but picked up by *Time Magazine* for the lay public. The doctors, pointing to a century of progress in making birth happier and more comfortable, saw natural childbirth as a step backward, an erosion of all that progress. To demonstrate their argument, they pictured women chatting over a game of bridge while they gossiped about childbirth. Formerly these women would have discussed the merits of different drugs in labor. Now, however, under this new reactionary influence, they might entertain one another with vivid details of an undrugged labor, including, the doctors wrote with a visible shudder, "the ecstasy of the unassisted expulsion of the placenta." The leader of this subversion of medical science was Grantly Dick-Read and his ideas. The doctors conceded there might be some slight benefit if reduction of fear enabled women to endure labor with smaller doses of drugs. And as utilized by a trained specialist, the theories might do no great harm. The potential harm lay in the way in which Read training hid other fears of childbirth, "deep seated anxieties . . . (about) increased responsibility, loss of personal freedom, economic hardships, and overcrowding of the home." Such worries, masked by what the doctors termed Read's "psychological lobotomy," could make childbirth more difficult.[12]

A few years later, the fears and motives of women who sought natural childbirth training were analyzed by a Boston obstetrician as part of a full-scale attack. In an article titled "The Medical Case against Natural Childbirth," co-authors Dr. Waldo Fielding and Lois Benjamin identified four types of failures commonly produced by Read training.

The first two were easily disposed of: one was the woman who simply dropped out of prenatal classes for a variety of reasons, and the second was the woman who found during labor that the reality was considerably different from the ideal promised in classes—the woman who opted for drugs when the pain was too great and the relaxation techniques useless. The third type of failure, with two possible sub-groups, was more interesting. In the first subdivision the woman, although suffering intensely, remained stoic and silent through labor because she wanted others to think of her as a success at undrugged birth. The second subtype shrieked and writhed her way through labor while stubbornly refusing drugs and afterwards insisted that birth had been a beautiful experience. "This woman causes doctors a great deal of concern because she covers up rather than dispels her conflict."

The fourth type of failure was the most distressing of all and resulted in the most sinister outcome. This was the damaged or disturbed woman, the very sort, according to the authors, most likely to be enthusiastic about natural birth. Psychiatrists disagreed on the origin of such inclination: some insisted it came from the desire to prove authentic femininity, while others declared the root was quite the opposite—a drive for power or "psycho-masculinity." No matter which, the obstetrician was left to worry about the "grave and permanent psychic harm" that came from allowing such disturbed women to attempt to give birth without drugs.[13]

From this viewpoint, a woman who entertained any idea about natural childbirth was a failure whether she managed to survive labor screaming or silent, or even if she had done nothing more than attend a few classes. The Fielding case was set in a larger context in which objections to medical interference such as routine anesthetics and episiotomy and low-forceps were argued and dismissed, but the main focus was on the suspected mental states of women advocates.

Even doctors who favored training for birth cast suspicious eyes on certain troublesome patients. One such doctor whose practice consisted mostly of natural childbirth candidates, said the majority were well-adjusted, but there was another 20 percent whom he labeled as "the pre-Serutan girls. They are the compulsives who wear Oxford shoes and walk into the office with a pad and pencil to write down exactly what you tell them—that's the compulsive neurotic group, the faddists."[14] Presumably mentally fit women didn't need to take notes in the consulting room.

In the same news article, Dr. C. Lee Buxton, Thoms' successor in the Yale program, admitted that the aim of providing an experience that was emotionally satisfying to the mother was not sufficient justification for a delivery method based on noninterference. "It must be a beneficial obstetrical technique (as well). . . . After all, there are an awful lot of things women want that they shouldn't have."[15]

Evidence that women were asking for what they wanted obstet-rically is generally missing during this period. A first-hand experience of prepared birth rarely appeared in the popular press. One, written by a doctor's wife who viewed her experience favorably, was published by *Parents' Magazine*. Another, in which an English woman dismissed the whole movement, appeared in *Mademoiselle* in 1962. "I believe," the latter wrote, "that childbearing at the moment is bedeviled with theory and absurdly complicated by self-consciousness. Some blame should, I think, rest on women's magazines which have a morbid obsession with parturition."[16] However, there is small record of women making strident demands, or any demands at all, either in obstetricians' waiting rooms or in the pages of the popular press. With one striking exception, the audible combatants were male experts.

## Marjorie Karmel

The exception was Marjorie Karmel, a beautiful young graduate of Bryn Mawr, actress, and fledgling playwright with her novelist husband, Alex. Her article, "A New Method of Painless Childbirth" was published in 1957 in a fashion magazine (*Harper's Bazaar*) after being rejected as too controversial elsewhere. The new method to which she referred had originated in the Soviet Union and migrated to France. It was at that time virtually unknown in the United States, although the Pope had given the method his qualified approval a year earlier. Marjorie's story began about the same time. In the midst of her first pregnancy and while on an ocean voyage to France, she read Read. Convinced that a birth during which she was awake and contributing was what she wanted, she set out to procure it in Paris. Some persistence brought the Karmels to the dim and heavily furnished consulting rooms of an older doctor, white-haired and jolly Fernand Lamaze. He asked what he could do for the young couple, and Marjorie, thinking her advanced state of pregnancy ought to provide the answer, responded that she had read Grantly Dick-Read.

Immediately Lamaze interrupted.

"Dr. Read's method is *accouchement sans crainte* (childbirth without fear); I give you *accouchement sans douleur* (childbirth without pain.) Are you interested?"[17] Naturally intrigued, Marjorie and Alex Karmel soon found themselves committed to a method designed to banish all the pain of bearing children. Marjorie learned there were other differences between Lamaze and Read. Whereas Read posed an idealized vision of motherhood in which women, in touch with their true natures, transcended fear and, therefore, pain, Lamaze offered a series of physical and mental exercises designed to change the perception of pain. Lamaze believed that conquering fear through knowledge and support as Read advised was only part of what was required. Women must also alter the patterns of perception that told them they were suffering. This revolution in perception would come about through newly conditioned reflexes which, instead of signaling pain, would signal the work of producing a child, and thus carry the woman through labor awake, aware, and in control of her own body.

This idea appealed to Marjorie as being more active and useful than Read's theories of transcendence. Her distaste for the mystical experience was shared by most other American women of the time. Two decades later a vision of childbirth as a transcendent experience was less likely to be dismissed as embarrassingly irrational, but in the late fifties, Lamaze techniques with their aura of scientific precision were much more acceptable. Marjorie soon began instruction in the method at the hands of Dr. Lamaze's *monitrice* and teacher, Madame Cohen, a woman of conviction who insisted that birth under the mother's control was good, even beautiful. To demonstrate, she showed her pupil photographs of women straining, their perineums slowly bulging with the head of the unborn child. Marjorie, whose fantasies of natural birth never included that particular view, was shaken, perhaps horrified, but still attracted. She stuck to the course, even after attending a film showing in vivid action the process of an undrugged birth, a view that shocked her so deeply she and Alex repaired to a corner cafe for cognac to aid in their recovery. Still, she persisted in learning breathing techniques for pushing when required and panting when not, all performed in the spirit of a competition.

The basis of the techniques came from the experiments of Pavlov and his famous salivating dog. Pavlov demonstrated that if an electric shock always preceded the offering of food, in time the dog no longer perceived the shock as pain, but rather as a signal of gratification to come. Similarly, other Russians reasoned, women might relearn how to accept the powerful uterine contractions of labor as a signal of the coming reward of birth. A prime experimentor, Mrs. N. Erofeeva, demonstrated that painful sensations rose from conditioned stimuli acting at the cortical level; as such they could be repressed by the intervention of new conditioning. According to Lamaze, her work provoked an English physiologist to exclaim, "Now I understand the psychology of martyrs!"[18]

Over the years, these theories were refined through further experimentation into a workable method for eliminating pain in childbirth, a method eventually so successful that the Russian government decreed its use mandatory in all maternity wards in 1959. That was the very year that Lamaze, a conventional French obstetrician, visited the country. Everywhere he saw the method in use, and in Leningrad he was permitted to watch a painless birth in its entirety.

> I had at the time thirty years of experience as an obstetrician. I had never been taught anything like this. I had never seen it, nor had I ever thought it could be possible. My emotional reaction was therefore all the stronger. I made a clean sweep of all preconceived ideas and, now an elderly schoolboy of sixty, I immediately decided to begin studying this new science.[19]

His middle-class patients back home rejected the new ideas, particularly as they had originated behind the Iron Curtain, and Lamaze lost much of his former practice which left him more time to refine the new techniques for use in *Maternité du Métallurgiste*, the clinic of the Metalworker's union where he was obstetrical chief. When it became apparent he would require more staff and some alteration in facilities, he applied to the French government for funds. Thus, what was known in France as the psycho-prophylactic (literally mind-prevention) method of controlling pain in birth, became a matter of public debate. People argued furiously over the value of an import tinged with the "godless materialism" of Russia, and the controversy grew so heated that it came to the attention of Pope Pius XII.

Early in 1956, the Pope presented a paper on the subject before a crowd of 700 obstetricians at the Vatican. Referring to the pain of birth as redefined by the new discoveries, he called it "real pain resulting from falsely interpreted causes." Sacred scripture did not forbid science to eliminate the sources of this pain, and its disappearance would decrease inducement to "commit immoral acts in the use of marriage rights," (presumably a reference to contraception). Furthermore, the bonds of motherly affection formed at birth would surely be enhanced if the woman were fully conscious.

However, the Pope warned, a Christian faced with a scientific discovery of this sort, especially one originating in a godless culture would be careful "not to admire it unreservedly and not to use it with exaggerated haste."[20]

Six months before the Pope gave his approval, Marjorie Karmel had successfully borne her first child in a Parisian hospital, *sans doleur*. After twenty-four hours of first-stage labor, she was finally ready to push the baby out as she had been instructed by Madame Cohen.

"Where previously everyone had spoken in soft and moderate tones in deference to my concentration, now there was a wild encouraging cheering section, dedicated to spurring me on. I felt like a football star, headed for a touchdown. My fans on the sidelines, Dr. Lamaze, Mme. Cohen, the midwife, the nurse, all exhorted me *POUSSEZ! POUSSEZ! POUSSEZ! POUSSEZ! CONTINUEZ! CONTINUEZ! CONTINUEZ! ENCORE! ENCORE!*"[21]

A few moments later she gave birth to a son. When she and Alex returned to New York a short time later, she was still fired with enthusiasm over the experience and longed to share it with friends. Most of them responded with a certain measure of hostility:

"I'm sure it works if you believe in it. . . . And if you think it's worth the trouble. . . . Some of us are braver than others. . . . But you have short easy labors. . . . You must have no nervous system . . . Having a baby is simple as pie *only* if you're not neurotic."[22]

Marjorie wrote the story of her Paris adventure and submitted it to a women's magazine where the editors gave the piece much thought but rejected it as too controversial; whether because it was concerned with childbirth or Russian theories, they did not say. By then Marjorie, pregnant again and unable to return to Paris, was trying to find a New York obstetrician willing to go along with Lamaze. The first attempt turned up a mature man with an excellent reputation and clientele. He declared himself on the side of drugless labor as intended by nature. "Out of a woman's suffering springs mother love," he said and wouldn't listen when Marjorie explained that suffering wasn't what she had in mind. The second doctor, a pixyish fellow, insisted first that she wasn't pregnant at all and couldn't be until he had straightened out her uterus; then discovering his mistake, said all would be just as she wished until the moment he put her out. The third try produced a younger man given to staring intently into her face while he questioned her in whispers. He informed her that the obstetrician's relationship with his patient was very like that in psychoanalysis. "To have valid meaning, there must be a transference; the doctor must be a sort of father image." He also called her by her first name, which she found as irritating as his therapeutic manner. Of course she was annoyed, Alex said, "One way first-name calling always means inequality—witness servants, children and dogs."[23]

Eventually she found a willing if not entirely convinced doctor. Feeling it was best to know the rules before attempting to breach them, Marjorie took a class in prepared childbirth at the hospital where she expected to give birth. The experience provided a good view of how natural childbirth was regarded in America in the late fifties. The class seemed geared to the lowest level of intelligence and highest level of fear among the pregnant women. After a long build-up to the pictures of birth they were going to see and warnings about their frank nature, Marjorie was dismayed to find the teacher displaying only the old MCA charts of sculptured models and not actual photographs of the baby bulging against the perineum which had so shocked and then reassured her in Mme. Cohen's class. When she protested to her doctor that she found much of the class instruction was bad conditioning, he responded that Americans did not take to doctrinaire and dogmatic training of the sort she had received in Paris.

"You know what psycho-prophylactic means don't you? . . . Brainwashing."

Marjorie said perhaps Lamaze training *was* a form of brainwashing in that it emptied the mind of destructive associations while providing tools that worked during labor. She was further dismayed by the doctor's somewhat embarrassed reaction when she showed him the birth photographs which had been included in a book written by Lamaze associate Dr. Pierre Vellay. It occurred to her that much of the way in which labor was managed in America had to do with prudery.

"For instance, all that draping and wrapping in the examining and delivery room. I couldn't believe it was all for the purpose of sterility. . . . I began to wonder if some of the attraction of anesthesia for both doctors and women didn't lie in the sop it offered to modesty."[24]

Although shaken by American attitudes that would make having a Lamaze birth difficult, Marjorie persevered, encouraged by stories from other women both here and abroad who had managed to retain some control over their labor. One friend had trained herself by studying Read on her own. In the delivery room, the anesthetist tried to force a mask on her face in spite of her vigorous protests, so she jabbed him in self-defense and broke off one of his teeth. Very shortly thereafter, she gave birth without drugs while everyone cheered except the anesthetist.

Marjorie's second labor was nearly as precipitate. Following a premature but only partial rupture of the amniotic sac, her obstetrician talked her into induction, assuring her there was very little difference between an induced labor and a spontaneous one. After fully puncturing the membranes, he began injecting ocytoxin periodically. "Each time I began to feel overconfident, Dr. Sedley returned with another shot. Off the contractions raced, and off I went after them."[25]

Nevertheless, Marjorie managed to stay in control, refusing all other interferences, including episiotomy and drugs offered just to "take off the edge." Within a short time her second child, a daughter, was born, and Marjorie had once again given birth *sans doleur.* Her own assessment was: "I do think of labor as a contest. And I think it is worth taking the trouble to win."[26]

This sort of spirit infused her article on natural childbirth which had finally been published in *Harper's Bazaar* a few months earlier. She wrote of the psycho-prophylactic method: "In the United States it is unknown even by name to all but a few obstetricians who pay attention to foreign developments, and is practiced nowhere. . . . It seems a pity that our country, usually so advanced in medicine, should have neglected something so important and beneficial!"[27]

That passage with its airy dismissal of all other advances in childbirth education irritated one reader, particularly because she herself had been involved in the American movement. Still, Elisabeth Bing was struck by the pragmatic aspects of the new technique, as Marjorie presented them, and was even more intrigued when a French visitor to Mt. Sinai referred to the method during a grand rounds tour of the hospital. At the same time, the first American book on the subject appeared—*Psychoprophylactic Preparation for Painless Childbirth* (Grune and Stratton, New York 1958)—written by a Cleveland doctor, Isadore Bonstein. After Elisabeth read this, she began casting about for funds that would enable her to go to Paris to study with Dr. Vellay. Then a woman came to her for childbirth training, a lively and inquisitive engineer expecting her second child. Elisabeth proposed that the woman try Lamaze instead of Read techniques for labor and the woman agreed, although she had only a week left to prepare. After the birth she called Elisabeth from her hospital bed saying the method had worked almost like magic and the rapid breathing especially had been a lifesaver.

The full story of Marjorie's adventures in both Paris and New York appeared as a book the following year entitled *Thank You, Doctor Lamaze*. Reading it, Elisabeth was totally won over. She wrote the publisher for an address and discovered the author was a neighboring New Yorker. The two women met and began a collaboration that was to profoundly influence childbirth education in the United States.

## ASPO—The American Society For Psychoprophylaxis in Obstetrics

Marjorie and Elisabeth decided immediately to create an organization for the promotion of Lamaze methods that would include physicians from the beginning as a means of influencing the profession. The first job was to convince a few leaders. Accordingly, they got hold of a French film, "Naissance," which had to be smuggled into the country to avoid seizure as pornography. They showed it to small groups of doctors, nurses, and midwives in the Karmels' elegant apartment. In the viewing and discussions which followed, various influential people were introduced to the principles of psychoprophylaxis in birth, among them Frederick Goodrich, author of *Natural Childbirth*; Hazel Corbin, director of the Maternity Center; and Benjamin Segal, an obstetrician who made a radical change in his life after learning about Lamaze. Instead of retiring, he launched a whole new practice based on Lamaze principles and, more importantly, agreed to become the first president of ASPO.

By 1960, the two women with others, including Elly Rakowitz, had turned up nine other doctors willing to join the enthusiastic Segal as physician founders of the organization. The idea was to establish a group partly composed of doctors, nurses, and physiotherapists who would bring ASPO practices into the prevailing system. To this end, the women behind the glossy front of professionals scurried about presenting films and workshops, serving coffee, and fueling discussions in their effort to convert doctors and nurses to the cause. All were independent women, but they deliberately tempered their assertiveness lest they scare off supporters. This strategy also influenced ASPO publications in which the presiding obstetrician was always granted full authority even in the matter of drugs.

"If he himself (the doctor) suggests medication, accept it willingly even though you don't feel the need for it. He undoubtedly has good reasons for his decision . . . "[28] Statements such as these appeared both in early and later texts for the psychoprophylactic method and were eventually sharply criticized by reformers. Still, it ought to be remembered that ASPO was founded in a time when nearly all reformists asked for a stamp of approval from doctors before presenting their theories to the public. So Bing, Karmel and Rakowitz were generally making use of an old strategy whereby the potential opponent would be disarmed by an offer of partnership in the campaign. The question of whether the tactic made Lamaze vulnerable to expropriation by medical professionals was not to surface for some time.

Following Lamaze's death, the society hosted a visit by Pierre Vellay who had succeeded to the leadership of the psychoprophylaxis movement in France. His presentation of a rigorous and carefully controlled discipline helped persuade at least a few American doctors that Lamaze methods were not at odds with good medicine nor in any way a hypnotic process, as some had charged. When Elisabeth made her pilgrimage to Paris, he acted as her host, inviting her to stay in his home and introducing her to his colleague, Dr. Zila Rennert, a refugee from Austria who was the major instructor in the method and a superb teacher, according to Elisabeth. As Mme. Cohen had done before her, Dr. Rennert carried on much of the important work of the movement, yet her name was almost unknown beyond the clinic, whereas Vellay as Lamaze's successor gained international recognition.

Elisabeth returned to New York eager to experiment with Lamaze techniques at Mt. Sinai. With Guttmacher's permission, she forged ahead in the face of even more hostility than before. This time the resentment, in more overt form than knowing glances and rude remarks, came from doctors who were used to compliant patients and not at all pleased to be confronted by women insisting on a Lamaze birth. The women who read Karmel's book asked hard questions at office visits and sometimes actually refused drugs during labor. Finally an obstetrician demanded of Guttmacher that Elisabeth be reprimanded for causing a rebellion among pregnant patients. He was not satisfied with Guttmacher's compromise offer of a warning in private but insisted on a public chastisement. Summoned to a grand rounds gathering with all the medical staff present, Elisabeth was asked to defend what some referred to contemptuously as the "lollipop method," a reference to common Lamaze advice about using hard candy during labor to ease dryness of the mouth.

The charges were mainly based on Elisabeth's use of *Thank You, Doctor Lamaze* which physicians, no doubt stung by Karmel's story of the three New York obstetricians, considered a wicked and unfair attack. Before Elisabeth could respond, supporters came to her defense and soon the two groups were arguing among themselves while she stood on the sidelines. After a hot debate, the medical staff concluded that Mrs. Bing could remain as childbirth educator at Mt. Sinai, but under no circumstances could she refer to the "objectionable book." For the remainder of her stay at the hospital the rule stayed in force, although inevitably during the course of a prenatal class, Bing managed to mention Marjorie's book.

Soon afterward Elisabeth moved to Flower and Fifth Avenue Hospital where her post was listed as clinical assistant professor which meant, she reported wryly, that she had an impressive title but not the salary allotted to someone called an "assistant clinical" professor.

In 1961 the ASPO bylaws were changed, splitting the organization into three divisions: one for doctors, a second for childbirth educators, and a third for parents. All three were to have equal representation on the board and equal voting rights, as Elisabeth and Marjorie had wanted from the beginning. The two women always worked well together. Elisabeth with her European elegance and restraint, and tall red-haired Marjorie with what Elly Rakowitz called a "dynamite" smile, and an ability to put others at their ease, made an excellent team for the Lamaze campaign. They collaborated on a small book of instructions called "The Red Book" by supporters, although the official title was *A Practical Training Course For the Psycho-prophylactic Method of Childbirth.* It had served as both a text for classes and a teaching manual for others who wanted to learn how to instruct parents. Now they were filled with fresh enthusiasm for the restructured ASPO, planning to organize members in each of the divisions for greater influence on local communities. But Marjorie's participation was cut short when it was discovered that she had breast cancer, the disease that had killed her mother.

After undergoing a radical mastectomy, Marjorie went to the Caribbean with her family where it was hoped she would recuperate. Already the mother of three small children, she became accidently pregnant again, and the cancer erupted anew. After the Karmels returned to New York, Marjorie's health swiftly declined. The illness of her friend brought back all Elisabeth's buried memories of the deaths of her father, mother, and second husband. "It was my first experience of being with someone I loved who was dying." Grief at her friend's death in March 1964, was eased by the knowledge that Marjorie believed she had completed her life's work in promoting Lamaze and co-founding ASPO. Even dying, Marjorie never gave up her smile.

After her death, Elisabeth was urged to update and popularize the "Red Book." Writing was difficult for her, especially working alone, and she did not complete *Six Practical Lessons For an Easier Childbirth* (Grosset and Dunlap) until 1967. As Alan Guttmacher predicted in his introduction to the book, it became a bible for parents involved in studying Lamaze. Since its first publication, the book has gone through nineteen printings and has been translated into German, French, Hebrew and Japanese. Since the enormous and continuing success of *Six Practical Lessons*, Elisabeth has published several more books: *A Birth in the Family* (1973), co-authored by Dr. Gerold Barrad; *Moving Through Pregnancy* (1975); and two on which she collaborated with California psychologist Libby Coleman. The first of these, *Making Love During Pregnancy* (Bantam, 1977) illustrated by David Passalacqua with explicit drawings of a pregnant woman and her partner making love, was rejected by one publisher because he thought it qualified as pornography and, following publication, was ignored by the usual publicity outlets in the United States. (Translated into French, German and Yugoslavian, it has sold well abroad.) From her old world view, Elisabeth felt the American response came from leftover Puritanism, a prudishness that sees the achievement of motherhood as saintly but does not wish to be reminded of the origin.

Again working with Libby Coleman, she wrote *Having a Baby after Thirty* (Bantam, 1980) which appealed to the increasing numbers of women who had postponed parenthood. "Never before have so many women been so effective in not having babies until they wanted them," the two women wrote in the introduction.[29] Personal experiences by both authors enlivened the pages with reassurance and advice for older mothers. "I stopped being self-conscious about being 'an old lady of 40,' because nobody else seemed to be bothered by it," Elisabeth wrote.[30]

Elisabeth Bing's career was linked with the growth of ASPO

across the country and with the rapidly growing popularity of Lamaze methods. In reviewing those early years, Elly Rakowitz wrote that "hospitals reluctantly creaked open their delivery rooms," first admitting fathers and eventually anyone the mother wanted with her during birth.[31] It was exhilarating to see Lamaze ideals percolate through the culture to a point where pregnant characters in a television drama might be found doing their exercises straight out of *Six Practical Lessons*, or the father, formerly treated as a distant and helpless observer, might be seen timing his wife's contractions during labor.

In time the term "Lamaze" came to cover a variety of conditions, some far removed from the doctrinaire training Marjorie Karmel had received from Mme. Cohen in 1955. Any of the general aims of natural childbirth: consciousness while giving birth, a minimum of medication, spontaneous as opposed to forceps delivery, prenatal education of the parents, and participation of the father, or all of these combined might be called "Lamaze" without including the specific principles of psychoprophylaxis. In fact, as time went on and Lamaze became more and more popular, some hospitals offered classes they called "Lamaze training," which were actually preparation for routine procedures in their maternity ward and delivery room. Parents might emerge from classes believing they were "doing Lamaze" when they had simply been indoctrinated into accepting that particular hospital's brand of labor management.

In time, Elizabeth, too, became less optimistic that doctors would accept a working relationship with their patients; they were too firmly indoctrinated with a belief that normal birth takes place only in retrospect. In the beginning, when Lamaze classes were mushrooming in every community, there seemed good reason to hope for major changes. Yet while reformers were looking to the future, the old quarrel about who should control birth was still rumbling along. Now and then a fresh combatant would enter the fray.

In 1952, anthropologist Ashley Montagu had protested hospital control, particularly for the sake of the newborn. "At a time when he needs his mother most, he is tagged, made antiseptic and taken away to a sterile room with all the other little criminals."[32] Echoing Dr. Neilsen's concerns of twenty years earlier, he declared that drugs given during labor had caused "thousands of children to become idiots and left thousands of others less bright than they otherwise would be." Montagu elaborated his case against routine hospital birth in an article for *Ladies' Home Journal* in 1956. "The hospital," he wrote, "tends to dehumanize the mother-child relationship, the very relationship out of which all humanity grows." Even on the basis of good medical practice, hospitals functioned to the detriment of the birthing woman. The three great dangers immediately after birth, Montagu noted, were hemorrhaging, failure of the placenta to separate, and failure of the uterus to return to normal. All these conditions could be forestalled by putting the newborn immediately to its mother's breast, an action that was considered inconvenient for hospital routine.

His solution was not only a return to home as the preferred place of birth, but a revival of the old birth helper, "the ancient and honorable calling of midwivery." Of course he hastened to add that he did not mean a resurrection of the ignorant granny of yore, but a new professional, the registered nurse midwife. "I foresee through this agency midwifery, medicine may begin once more to be humanized in its devotion to humanity, as it was before specialization set in in its present extreme form."[33]

Readers' response to the Montagu proposals was generally negative. "I couldn't disagree more. . . . How much simpler and more restful to be in a hospital where babies are an accepted business," commented one. "Why should a woman want her family to share in her labor moans and groans and so on? Why should she prefer a midwife to a well-qualified M.D. whom she has known and trusted for nine months? Doctor Montagu's advantages seem ridiculous to me." Another woman was indignant at the implication that pregnant women, so dependent and grateful for safe delivery, developed an unhealthy fantasy relationship with their obstetricians. "I have the utmost respect for my obstetrician, but I did not fall in love with him! The grocery boy delivers the groceries, and most of us gals manage not to mix him up with the wonderful guy who foots the bills!" A woman who signed herself as "loyal, disgruntled reader," declared that she was furious. "If men don't stop writing articles telling women what to do about childbirth, I'm going to burst!"[34]

This understandable sentiment had no effect, of course, on the continuing dispute over who was to be in control of birth. In addition to doctors, anthropologists, psychologists and journalists, another sort of expert took up the argument in the person of Sloan Wilson, bestselling novelist who published the tale of his second wife's pregnancy and labor in *Harper's*, June 1964.

"Now as I was about to become a father again, new theories

about childbirth were being talked about in bars and I had to find the best way of doing things."[35]

Accordingly, he read Marjorie Karmel's book and Karen Pryor's on breastfeeding and was soon convinced by what he described as an "exuberant, earthy philosophy which glorified the act of birth as the supreme moment in life, and celebrated nursing as a mystic communion between mother and child. . . . " The optimum circumstances were those old standbys of natural childbirth advocates—the father's presence during labor and delivery, no drugs unless absolutely necessary, encouragement for breastfeeding and rooming in. These conditions, he was assured by the informant at his local bar, would produce a healthful child, one less likely as an adult to smoke or drink too much or to build hydrogen bombs in preference to schools and hospitals for the poor. Wilson presented his requests in writing and received qualified assurances from a clearly long-suffering obstetrician that the birth would occur as he wished—if all went well. Unfortunately, all did not go well in spite of classes and exercises, and following a long, stalled labor, delivery was performed under complete anesthesia with forceps and episiotomy. Reflecting that in an earlier time his wife might have died, Wilson concluded, "When things mysteriously go wrong, the American way of birth is nothing to be regarded with contempt . . . (it) is much derided these days by male intellectuals, but women of all backgrounds, I find, speak rather softly about it, at least after they have had their first child."[36]

Wilson's humble retreat from criticism of medical obstetrics was not enough to mollify one doctor (Allan C. Barnes, chief ob-gynecologist at Johns Hopkins). Proposing a change in title to "The Man in the Grey Flannel Scrub Suit" and a shift from the wife's condition of pregnancy to that of diseased gall bladder, Barnes rewrote the scenario. His narrator, mulling over his responsibility for choosing the anesthesia for his wife's surgery, concludes, "Before arranging the appointment with the doctor when I would tell him my decision in this matter, however, I set out for the corner bar where the best advice on these subjects can always be obtained."[37]

## Cruelty on the Maternity Wards

Outrageous as Wilson's presumption seemed, it was clear that neither Barnes, nor Montagu, nor any of the other experts arguing about how childbirth should be managed gave much weight to the opinion of the chief participants in the process—the women themselves. They may all have believed with Buxton at Yale that "there are an awful lot of things women want that they shouldn't have" and, therefore, they should generally be ignored. In that era of submission, it was easy to discard women's opinions about birth because with few exceptions they were simply not heard, at least publicly, and few knew how women regarded their birth experiences. An exception was an outpouring in the pages of *Ladies' Home Journal* during 1958, prompted by a single letter from a registered nurse who dared not sign her name for fear of reprisal. She wrote to complain of cruelty she had witnessed on maternity wards and the *Journal* invited readers to comment. In the resulting flood of letters which continued all through 1958, charges made by "Registered Nurse" were corroborated and several new ones added.

The first complaint was that women were strapped hand, shoulder, and foot, on the delivery table and left sometimes for hours. Many correspondents agreed, often with grim details:

"With leather cuffs strapped around my wrists and legs, I was left alone for nearly eight hours until the actual delivery."

"My obstetrician wanted to get home for dinner. When I was taken to the delivery room my legs were tied way up in the air and spread as far apart as they would go. . . . when I was securely tied down I was left alone."

"My baby arrived after I had lain on the table in delivery position for nearly four hours."

Nurses whom the *Journal* editors consulted on this point generally insisted all was done for the mother's safety and even comfort: "Registered Nurse probably never had a baby or she would know that the lithotomy position is quite comfortable during labor," responded one nurse.

The second charge, that births were commonly held back to wait the doctor's arrival, was echoed by nearly half the letter writers and drew few denials from staff.

"I was strapped on the delivery table. My doctor had not arrived and the nurses held my legs together. I was helpless and at their mercy. They held my baby back until the doctor came into the room. She was born while he was washing his hands."

" . . . when the nurse finally examined me she sent for another nurse to call the doctor immediately while she strapped my legs together and gave me ether until the doctor arrived. . . . (he) had to come eight miles."

"The doctor ... went out to make a house call. One hour later my legs were released in the stirrups and held together by a nurse who sat on my knees, up on the delivery table, mind you, because the baby was coming so fast."

"The granddaughter of a neighbor is hopelessly brain-injured because nurses tied the mother's legs together to slow down the birth until the doctor arrived."[38]

Physicians whom the editors consulted on this charge said there was no defense for holding back a birth until the doctor arrived. However, they agreed that nurses who tied legs together, who sat on women, could not be blamed because they had to carry out orders or lose their positions, no matter what their own judgment of the situation might be.

There were other accusations against nurses: charges of callous treatment and verbal abuse, of laboring women being told they'd had their fun and now must suffer for it. Correspondents who were nurses themselves acknowledged hearing such remarks and sometimes from nurses who had also borne children. One woman wrote: "I believe that there exists among nurses a definite hostility toward women in childbirth ... There seems to be a feeling that a woman in childbirth has brought her troubles on herself and so deserves no kindness."[39]

Whether nurses were actually hostile to maternity patients, *Journal* readers certainly charged them with cruelty, along with doctors and other staff members. One woman reported that her female anesthetist, in an attempt to get her to stop yelling, had asked repeatedly, "Do you want a misfit or a dead baby? You're killing it every time you yell for the doctor. ... "[40]

Perhaps as damaging as the verbal abuse was the women's sense that they were being treated as little more than objects in a system designed primarily for the efficient removal of infants in the quickest way possible. Medical authorities admitted that with so many women being delivered it was possible care could be mechanical at times, although they felt that could easily be remedied by hospital administrators.

Another charge few doctors or nurses took the trouble to deny was that women were left alone for long frightening periods during the first stage of labor. One woman wrote of being abandoned an entire night. "I felt exactly like a trapped animal and I am sure I would have committed suicide if I had had the means. ... " Doctors conceded this charge was often accurate; abandonment occurred not because of intention, but again because there were so many women to be delivered and so few staff members to attend them. A nurse could not afford to sit with a woman during the long first stage of labor when nothing much was happening, any more than "Tell-Me-Doctor" Sanford could. The *Journal* responded that women ought to be allowed the company of their husbands or of some relative or friend, as it used to be before childbirth was turned into a "medical mystery conducted in secret."[41]

Letters continued to pour in the *Journal* offices through the year. In December 1958, the editors printed another article with excerpts from subsequent correspondence and a list of recommendations for reform. Heading the article was the full text of a letter from somewhere on the west coast—a chronicle of abuse and neglect during birth. The letter was written by a woman whose child, then nine years old, had recently been diagnosed as retarded. The parents, searching for the cause, had returned to the circumstances of their son's birth:

> I still cringe when I remember the night Danny was born. I was in a large hospital in a well-known city, and I had a reputable and popular obstetrician. At ten-thirty a nurse told me that my baby had crowned and that he had black hair. Then she called the doctor. When the doctor didn't arrive in time, they stopped me from giving birth by holding my legs together until I was given anesthesia. The time of delivery on the birth record is two-thirty A.M. What happened during those three and more hours when I was held under anesthesia is only now evident. When I first saw Danny he was asleep. For several days it was almost impossible to rouse him long enough to nurse. On each side of his head there was a swollen purple bruise, but the obstetrician denied he had used instruments. "The birth," he said, "was free of all complications." . . . It would not be true to say that we haven't felt anger. But against whom do we direct it? . . . This fall we are expecting another child. We have arranged to drive twenty miles to the only hospital in our city that allows husbands to be with their wives during delivery. . . . From my heart I appeal to all parents: the responsibility for careful delivery of your unborn child rests on you. . . . Let us not produce more children who, for the sake of a few hours of convenience, must travel through life with one part of their minds unresponsive.[42]

## Lester Hazell: Getting What You Want

The call for parents to assume some of the responsibility for birth was an exception in a culture whose members, particularly women, had been advised for years to abdicate in favor of experts. But

Danny's mother was not the first woman to decide, usually in reaction to an unhappy experience, that she wanted more say in how the next birth would be managed. One such woman, Lester Hazell, destined to become a prime mover in the cause of childbirth reform, was converted after the birth of her first son in a Washington D.C. hospital in 1954.

As she later wrote (*Commonsense Childbirth*, 1969), she, along with most other American women, had expected the hospital and doctor to have the baby for her and reckoned the process for a healthy young woman like herself would be a simple matter. Instead it was a nightmare. When the delivery date was two weeks past, Lester's doctor recommended induction. After many hours of contractions, an attempt was made at caudal anesthesia. When it failed, Lester was given nembutal producing the nightmarish quality of "twilight sleep." Eventually, a forceps delivery was performed while she was under gas. Her first reaction to her bruised son with his head purplish and misshapen from the instruments was one of shocked dismay. Anxious to make up for the poor start, she was forced to wait for twenty-four hours before the child was brought to her for a first feeding. Then it was the wrong child.

"This isn't my baby. I saw mine in the delivery room and this isn't my baby!"

"Oh, honey," the nurse said, "you just don't remember. Here, take your baby and be a good girl."

But Lester continued to refuse the strange infant and when the nurse checked its bracelet, she discovered she did have the wrong one. Another baby boy born at the same time had been placed in the wrong crib, which would have been a minor concern except that the Hazell baby had an injury, probably correctable at birth but irremediable by the time the mix-up was discovered.

Lester was so distraught over these events that when her husband Bill took her and Jonathan home, she was capable of no more than sitting and rocking the baby in her arms. Bill Hazell was also disturbed at what should have been a joyous occasion. Instead it had meant for him thirty hours in a waiting room outside the labor suite, not knowing what had happened to his wife. Once Lester rocked herself and Jonathan back to composure, she decided to make certain such events could never happen again. She read all she could find on birth and talked with other women about their experiences. Later she wrote that had she done the same study before Jonathan's birth that she did afterward, the mix-up and the worsening of the slight injury would never have happened. So it was, in fact, partly her responsibility. With better preparation, "I would have known how to have my baby myself without forceps or drugs, and I would have picked a different doctor and hospital."[43]

These convictions, unusual in a young woman of the nineteen fifties, were typical of Lester who had seemingly known all her life when there was a remedy to be gained in taking action and when there was none. She was born in 1928, named for her father Lester Dessez, a career officer in the Marines, then a captain and later a general. Her mother Mary was a beautiful and delicate woman who hadn't a notion of how to raise her child. Lester's first memory of her was as a woman weeping in a doorway while she herself lay in a crib, also weeping. Lester felt she knew from that moment that she'd have to care for herself in order to survive.

When the baby was six months old, Mary Dessez was told she had to give her solid foods. Baby Lester spat them out and would have nothing but breastmilk. The pediatrician insisted and Mary, desperate over her failure to nourish her baby in the prescribed manner, put the child in a boarding home where she would be forced to eat. Contemporary response to such a solution of an infant eating problem is horror; however, in the twenties and thirties, mothers were advised that a rigid regularity was best for baby. Discipline led to a happy well-adjusted child, whereas indulgence of any sort tended to produce "little tyrants."

Far from being happy or even resigned, Lester went into a decline in the boarding home and stopped eating almost entirely. Finally Mrs. Dessez was told to come for her daughter lest the baby slip further into an infant despair now called marasmus. At the sight of her mother, Lester smiled for the first time in two months and reached out her arms. Weeping with remorse, Mary carried her child home to manage however she could. When Lester's father who'd been absent during the entire period returned, he took his wife to task for giving way to the pediatrician, and Mary found herself caught between her husband's beliefs in the emotional needs of children and the doctor's scientific theories on nutrition. She never understood what was best to do. Lester, with life-long confidence in her own perceptions, said of her mother: "There was a piece missing and it couldn't be helped. It was a fact like the sun and the rain. You don't get angry with the sun and the rain."

After several years as a member of the Marine Honor Guard at the White House, Captain Dessez was assigned to the French War

College, and the family moved to Paris when Lester was six. They returned to the United States in 1937; two years later, Mary Dessez gave birth to a second daughter. By then Lester had found a photographic essay on the birth of a baby in *Life Magazine*. The pictures were shockingly graphic for that period and caused a furor. In many homes the issue was hidden lest children see it and be damaged by the sight of an infant emerging from the mother's vagina. But the Dessez parents had no such strictures. Lester studied the pictures for hours and decided they showed an event that was both wonderful and awful. She longed to have a baby of her own some day and often brought home neighborhood children to mother, some toddlers so large their fat legs dangled around her ankles. After her sister Jeanne was born, there was no need to bring home stray babies. Mary Dessez, no more confident in her skills as a mother than she had been eleven years earlier, returned from the hospital and offered Jeanne to her older daughter. "I hope you can raise her."

During Captain Dessez' next tour of duty on Samoa, there were servants to help with the housework and the baby, and Lester rode down island roads to a convent school. This pleasant life ended abruptly in the summer of 1941 when Mary Dessez discovered a lump in one breast and had a radical mastectomy at Tripler Navy Hospital in Honolulu. After hearing a gloomy diagnosis which promised his wife no more than five years of life, and seeing his children settled in a boarding house, Captain Dessez returned to his post. His advice for Lester was that which he gave himself and his subordinates in the Marines. She must "pull up her socks and go on."

Not yet thirteen, Lester was left to comfort her despairing mother and care for the little one. She felt the end of the world had come those late summer days but that things were as they were and could not be changed, so she did as her father advised and soldiered on. The boarding house owner agreed to look after Jeanne while Lester visited her mother and later when she accompanied her to a series of radiation treatments. When Mary Dessez was finally released, having undergone all the treatment available, Lester took charge of seeing that the three of them got safely back to the States. After an exhausting flight to Washington D.C. where an aunt finally relieved her of total responsibility, she returned again to being, at least part of the time, a school girl.

Lester moved into adolescence with relative ease and good humor, enjoying an unusually friendly and honest relationship with her mother. Although cancer was ultimately to kill Mary Dessez in 1956, she was then in a period of remission and showed an unexpected talent for dealing with a teenager, teaching her to sew and answering sexual questions freely. Lester graduated with honors from Woodrow Wilson High School and worked her way through George Washington University, majoring in French literature, while living at home and caring for her little sister. After graduation in 1949, she followed her current boy friend, a medical student, to Georgetown University Hospital. As a medical technician there, she helped set up a pioneer kidney dialysis machine and participated in the first Papanicolau screening program for detecting cervical cancer.

In June 1951, she married Bill Hazell, the son of family friends, who had a physics degree from Harvard and was working on a master's in industrial psychology. After their first child, Jonathan, was born in 1954, the Hazells were increasingly involved in educating themselves and other young parents for birth. They had formed a group with other couples to improve birth management in local hospitals, and from this grew an organization called Parent and Child which sponsored natural childbirth classes in the Washington D.C. area. Because of her hospital work, Lester, with Jonathan in tow, had been sent to New York for a course at the Maternity Center where she learned how to teach the Read method.

Across the country, other groups of parents similarly galvanized were also organizing. In the early fifties, Virginia Larsen's students had formed the Association for Childbirth Education (ACE) in Seattle for training teachers and providing classes in childbirth preparation. They also advocated breastfeeding and rooming-in, as well as other components of a birth shared by both parents. However, they took care to explain that they weren't attacking medical management of birth, nor the doctors right to control, but only urging modifications. Even before organizing, they had asked the advice of a number of doctors in various specialities. In an article on the ACE for *Ladies' Home Journal*, one of the founding mothers is quoted: "From the very first, we have very much wanted professional people working with us — and not under the misapprehension that we were opposing existing systems of obstetrical care."[44] Actually the group did oppose some common practices on maternity wards and delivery rooms, but since their hope was to achieve change by first gaining the respect of physicians and staff, they tended to blunt any outright criticism — just as

ASPO in the same period intended to revolutionize attitudes toward labor by first converting obstetricians to their cause.

The same reluctance to criticize medical practice in face of public reverence for the profession prevailed nearly everywhere in the fifties and sixties. All campaigns for reviving midwifery were accompanied by the disclaimer that Montagu used: the new midwife would be a certified professional and always subordinate to the specialist in charge. No one wanted a revival of the old-time independent practitioner whom the AMA had succeeded in eliminating in the early years of the century. Nevertheless, through all these citizen movements ran a thread of radicalism, of revolt against medical control. Lester, who had always seen herself as standing to one side of the culture in which she lived, moved slowly but steadily away from received ideas toward new and perhaps daring possibilities.

When her second child was due, she and Bill were ready to try out some of these possibilities. They found a physician who would allow Bill's presence during the entire labor and delivery, and a hospital willing to permit rooming-in. Lester, in a standard hospital gown, her streaked blonde hair hanging to her waist, lay half-propped in her husband's arms while she labored unaided by any drugs or instruments. The birth resulting in a second boy, Jeremy, set a precedent in the hospital. Afterward, curious staff members kept dropping by Lester's room to watch an infant who didn't cry like all the others newborns in the central nursery. As a result, the administration began to loosen its policies and allow similar freedom to those parents who wanted it.

In 1959, Hazel Cobin as head of the Maternity Center Association had invited representatives from groups like Parent and Child in nine cities to come to a conference in New York to discuss their common problems in organization and programming. Out of this first gathering emerged the International Childbirth Education Association (ICEA), a federation of thirty different parent groups spread across the nation. The first national meeting, held in Milwaukee in 1960, affirmed a mutual belief in family-centered birth and a conviction that birth belonged to the parents and not the hospital (although at the time no one was radical enough to suggest that the hospital was not the best place for birth). The ICEA also advocated the cluster of conditions always favored by natural or prepared childbirth enthusiasts, but there was a fresh element in its philosophy—an emerging strain of consumerism. In an article in *Redbook* (July 1962), representatives of the new federation complained of overcrowded doctors' offices and hospitals, of busy obstetricians who gave little time for support and reassurance, of too few nurses on labor wards. While still deferring to the obstetrician's final authority, members felt that they had a right to full information about the birth process offered in classes geared to their intelligence level. The crusading spirit of ICEA was expressed in a vision of birth as a profound experience for both husband and wife and in a hope that the effect of ICEA ideals would be as revolutionary as the introduction of anesthesia had been a century earlier.

This spirit led members at the first meeting to debate whether professionals had any place in the federation at all. The point was energetically argued while health professionals like Dr. Virginia Larson and Margaret Gamper were told to wait outside the meeting hall. In the resulting vote they were granted membership under the unifying vision of ICEA's motto: "Parents and professionals working together to provide parents with the knowledge of alternatives to make an informed choice." In spite of this stated alliance and the number of professionals invited to serve as consultants, among them Margaret Mead and Ashley Montagu, the work of ICEA member groups was done largely by parent activists.

An early professional member and later director-at-large was Flora Hommel who had made the film "Naissance." Like Marjorie Karmel, Hommel had been a patient of Dr. Lamaze in Paris. She returned to America to teach psychoprophylaxis in Detroit and insisted on titling her ICEA group The Childbirth Without Pain Education Association despite criticism that it led to unrealistic expectations. She identified childbirth reform as a feminist struggle and invited feminists from all over the country to speak at her conferences in Detroit.

Another professional member was Tom Brewer, the ardent and radical obstetrician who has laid the blame for toxemia and other morbid conditions of pregnancy on malnutrition. Virginia Larsen and Carolyn Mann Rawlins were two other physicians who went against the obstetrical grain by helping to organize ICEA while conducting education and support groups for parents in their homes and offices. A number of such people with varying programs for change came together under the ICEA banner in the shared conviction that each mother and father was entitled to the sort of birth they thought right for them as a couple, as well as safe for their baby.

This philosophy, radical at center but always accepting individual variation, suited Lester Hazell exactly. From her earliest days in the reform movement, her plan had been to teach others not what they should have for their own good, or would have imposed on them willy-nilly, but how to get what they themselves wanted.

When their third child was due, Lester and Bill decided what they wanted was a home birth. They considered the possibility and began to prepare for it without actually deciding until they heard that a staphylococcic infection was making the rounds of newborn nurseries in Washington. Then it was determined: the next Hazell child would be born in the family home. During a long first stage labor, Lester baked bread and visited with her sister Jeanne who was also pregnant. Lester took to her bed early in the evening while her two small sons wandered in and out in pajamas. Friends were gathered, watchful and supportive, but there was no doctor; the Hazells were on their own.

Late in the evening, Lester entered a state of anxiety, wondering whether she were doing the right thing after all. Bill sustained his wife as he guided her with gentle teasing and encouragement through transition, the most difficult part of labor. She recovered her trust in the process as she began to push. The amniotic sack had not broken, and Bill Hazell could see it glistening as it bulged against the opening with each push. He punctured it, and soon the child's head was born, eyes open and looking about. When the whole baby emerged, Bill laid the little girl on his wife's breast. One friend was so overcome at seeing the birth that she heaved herself with relief into a frail rocker that promptly collapsed under her weight. Another friend laughed and then another, and soon everyone in the room was whooping, tears running down their cheeks in celebration of the new child who was to be Mary, her grandmother's namesake.

A year after Mary was born, the Hazells crossed the continent to California, and there Lester spent the next few years writing her guide for women in childbirth. She met a family doctor, Fred Fry, who delivered babies at home and began to accompany him as an assistant in Big Sur where a group of early hippies lived off the land. Lester attended about a dozen births there, sometimes catching the baby herself. She and Bill were teaching childbirth education again, urged by local parents who wanted training in natural childbirth. By that time, Lamaze as a method was widely known, and Lester made use of its appeal, calling her classes "modified Lamaze." Actually, the content was less specific instruction in breathing and more an attitude emphasizing serenity during pregnancy and birth. Accompanying the philosophy was an unswerving view of the pregnant woman and her partner as consumers. Health care, Lester insisted, was a service like any other, and people needed to shop around in order to find value for money.

In 1968 the Hazells went to Anaheim, California, for the Western Conference of the ICEA, one of four regional gatherings alternating with the international conference every other year. This was their first appearance as co-presidents, and they came to the rostrum in a time of high excitement, of faith that good maternity care could be made available to everyone in the nation, including those who could not pay. Then less than ten years old, the federated groups of the ICEA were proliferating in a country still committed to the ideals of Lyndon Johnson's Great Society.

Dispatching their three children across the road to Disneyland, the Hazells chaired meetings and hosted the handful of interested physicians who came to speak to a hall filled with parents, their infants in slings, backpacks, baskets, and strollers; their toddlers crawling on the floor through the forest of chairs. Veteran educators like Elisabeth Bing and Rhondda Hartman taught workshops in methods they had developed, and Pierre Vellay, the keynote speaker, presented his theories in French while Lester translated.

The audience was composed of lay people and professionals from all over the western region, eager to hear and spread the new philosophy of family-centered childbirth and consumer rights in health care. A growing awareness of those rights was merging with the human potential movement that had begun in California. Lester and Bill, in keeping with the new techniques, discussed the effects of body language, and Lester headed a workshop on the use of encounter groups in childbirth education. Shortly after the conference, the attractive couple, seen by many as forming the ideal ICEA family, changed their lives, moving into cramped student housing in Berkeley while Bill worked on a Ph.D. in Public Health and Lester studied anthropology.

By the time Bill Hazell finished his degree and the family moved to prosperous Marin County, Lester's book *Commonsense Childbirth* was in its first publication. She characterized it as a "cookbook" for labor and also a "polemic which is based on more than a decade of wading through the quagmire of American birth practices."[45] The core of the cookbook consisted of data Lester had summarized from observing hundreds of labors. At each labor, she had carefully noted not only the woman's response in detail and how responses changed from one stage to the another, but how all followed a general pattern. From this she constructed a description of what labor feels like, step by step, and how an attendant can best support the laboring woman at any given time. In the years since its first appearance, this unique documentation of labor and birth from a woman's point of view has remained remarkably instructive and touching. The entire book is infused with a humane concern for mother and child, combined with tough insistence on the rights and responsibilities of the parents. "We tend to act as if we were slaves to our present system of obstetrics. Yet none of us are. . . . it is parents themselves who must not only provide the impetus for change but must set the direction which change must take. . . . Emancipation lies not in escape from our destiny as parents but in control of that destiny."[46]

The book and her master's degree completed, Lester went to work as a rehabilitation counselor in a facility called The Center for Special Problems, in San Francisco. Among her clients were former inmates of state mental institutions currently turned back to communities, exconvicts, burned out drug users, and the sexually confused and exploited. In addition to using the new techniques of encounter and group therapy, Lester seemed to be carrying on her father's philosophy that people be taught how to pull up their socks and go on. By then Lester and Bill had been working in the midst of the birth reform movement for nearly twenty years, concentrating on the beginning of life. Now they were to confront the closing of life in the death of a child.

Shortly after midnight on Easter Sunday, 1974, Jeremy Hazell came in from attending a movie with his girl friend and asked for the car so he could drive her home. Lester stood in the hall, keys jangling as she handed them to him, and a shadow of premonition passed over her. Ten minutes later, the girl telephoned to say there had been an accident with the car. Jeremy had been thrown out across the road and now was being taken to Marin General Hospital. Lester and Bill drove their pick-up swiftly through deserted streets. While waiting for a traffic light, they saw a huge star fall across the sky, trailing pale fire as it went. At the hospital they found Jeremy living only by virtue of machinery; his brain was hopelessly damaged. For a few minutes they watched the equipment that kept his heart beating and lungs breathing. They talked quietly alone and then asked the doctors to pull the plugs, and Jeremy died with his parents holding his hands, his spirit borne away, Lester believed, with the falling star. "It was a glorious star."

During the next five days, the Hazell home overflowed with friends and relatives come not only to mourn death, but to celebrate a life. Pots of food bubbled on the stove, and Jeremy's friends gathered in small knots to tell again the story of the accident and to wonder how it could have happened. Jeanne arrived to help her sister while Lester comforted friends who grieved because they did not know how to comfort her. She and Jeanne acknowledged the pain of their absent and ailing father, the old Marine who wished, if his grandson had to die, he could have fallen in Vietnam while serving his country.

Lester felt very clear in her belief that Jeremy had moved from one stage of existence to another without a backward glance, just as he'd leaped into life as a child. She did not quarrel with his death, nor rail against it, nor deny it. You do not get angry with the wind and the rain. Once, alone briefly on the terrace, she saw a vision of Jeremy looking down on her from the roof. Several years earlier he had worked an entire day preparing a surprise which, to her horror, turned out to be his taking a running jump from the roof, flying over the pavement and diving into three feet of water in the pool. She had forbidden him to ever try the trick again. Now she saw him laughing and teasing her. Could he jump once more? "No dice," she said firmly, and Jeremy, laughing still, faded in the sunlight.

Early the last morning, Lester and Bill slipped out of the sleeping house and drove up the slopes of Mt. Tamalpais, a long peak overlooking the Golden Gate. In a meadow they scattered Jeremy's ashes to ocean winds and then went home for the final celebration where friends and family paid homage to their son with rock and folk music and eulogies. Fourteen-year-old Mary read an essay Jeremy had written about his mother's heirloom clock. When he realized it had been ticking long before he was born, before his father and even his grandfather were born, he had been chilled by the recognition of his own mortality, but then he was comforted by the thought of the clock ticking through all those lives and beyond. Now the clock still ticked, and Jeremy at seventeen was dead.

Three weeks later the Hazells flew with Mary and Jonathan to Tampa, Florida, where Lester was scheduled to make an address on birth at an ICEA convention. Instead she talked about death while childbirth educators, parents, doctors and nurses sat hushed and weeping. In a lowpitched but unbroken voice, she spoke

spontaneously of her son. "He was a remarkable piece of consciousness, a boy with a third eye, and a sense that made him sensitive to
the needs of us all. Now he is gone. . . . I am grateful to have known
him. . . . Unless you accept death, you cannot fully know birth."[47]

Back home in Corte Madera in the aftermath of tragedy, the
Hazell's marriage gradually disintegrated. Lester took an apartment
in San Francisco with Mary, returned for six months to the family
home, then finally decided to leave for good, taking only her
clothes and a few treasures, among them the grandfather clock.
Divorced in 1978 after twenty-seven years of marriage, Lester in
her fiftieth year struck out truly on her own for the first time in her
life.

Like others leaving the security of a marriage, she had to break
away from the image of herself as ideal wife and mother and
acknowledge that she was a single woman. For many in the childbirth
movement, a divorce had meant moving on, not from anything
actually said, but because of a conspiracy of silence around the fact
of broken marriages. In some ICEA and ASPO groups, due to the
emphasis on husband and wife sharing in childbirth, there was an
unspoken belief that a happy birth experience was insurance against
the possibility of divorce.

Lester Hazell was rare in remaining in the movement after she left
her husband and, more startlingly, her children who stayed with
their father in the security of the Corte Madera home. In the
eighties as a member of the part-time faculty at UC Medical Center,
she found among her students other women floundering in divorce
shock. These women, fledgling nurse midwives, not only had to
recover their self-respect; they had to acquire enough confidence and
fortitude to make independent judgments about clinical matters
and to stand up to doctors. Lester's old ability to respond to need,
together with her new perspective, made her an ideal mentor.

# THREE

# The Decline and Ressurrection of Breastfeeding 1900-Present

## Summer Illness

> Consider that for millions of years mammals had been breastfeeding. Then in just a fraction of a moment in time the human animal changed this. We just turned off the breast! . . . The great changeover, this take-over by the cow, began in America at the turn of the twentieth century and took but a few decades. Its roots, however, reach back more than a hundred years into the industrial revolution. . . . The bottle suddenly took on a special aura which went far beyond its function. It stood for modernity, and 'modern' in America meant 'good.' It symbolized liberation.[1]

This assessment by anthropologist Dana Raphael offers a fresh perspective on what has been referred to as the greatest uncontrolled experiment in history—the abandonment of the lactating female breast for a glass or plastic bottle, and the complicated human nipple for a rubber cap pricked with holes. Since the industrial revolution there have been many other radical alterations in ancient ways of caring for ourselves and our children, but no other was embarked on wholesale with such untested faith that the new way was better.

Until the turn of the century, the child of a woman unable or unwilling to breastfeed usually had one hope of survival, and that was the proximity of another lactating woman. Called "wet nurses," their numbers flourished most in times and places of sharp class distinction where an abundance of poor mothers could make a bare living by selling their milk to wealthier women who for some reason (often an excess of delicacy and refinement) did not nurse their infants.

In 1748, Dr. William Cadogan published a survey for the Governors' Foundling Hospital in London in which he estimated that less than 5 percent of affluent women were willing to nurse their children.[2] This pattern also prevailed in the American South before the Civil War when many privileged children nursed at the breasts of black women who were the property of their parents. Not all nurslings fared so well, as Dr. Judith Wertman has pointed out in her research on nutrition. If a family could not afford to give bed and board to a wet nurse, the babies might be farmed out to an unknown place in the country where they risked malnutrition, infection, and, if the wet nurse was inclined to sedate the baby with alcohol, drunkenness.[3]

Through the centuries various substitutes for breast milk, known as pap, were concocted. F. H. Richardson, a physician who has analyzed breastfeeding trends, notes the ingredients for some paps in use in the eighteenth and nineteenth centuries. One called "panada" was made of bread crumbs boiled in milk or broth, while "caudle" was made of bread, sugar, and spices laced with wine or ale. Infant food was also provided by the milk of domestic animals: asses, mares, goats and cows.

Nevertheless, until late in the nineteenth century breast milk was indispensable for the survival of infants. Then doctors began to look seriously for a substance with which to successfully "hand feed" infants. Richardson noted that "analyzing human milk and trying to concoct a substitute for it was a fascinating pursuit. But attempts to 'modify' the milk of the horse, goat, and cow all failed to make the grade, no matter how scientists added lactic acid, various kinds of sugars, or diluted it and boiled it. The mortality still remained high."[4]

Bottle or hand feeding had been launched when doctors discovered that boiling animal milk made it digestible for human babies. There was still the problem of milk storage in homes that mostly lacked any form of refrigeration. Those who could afford iceboxes bought ice twice a week from an iceman; those who couldn't depended solely on an aircooled cupboard or windowsill. Jane Addams, founder of the first settlement house in America, in a study on the relationship between disease and the bulk sales of milk, described the usual circumstances of trade in the city. "The milk wagon stopped in the fly-infested street to measure pint quantities of milk into a buyer's jar. The ladle used was seldom washed and always exposed."[5]

Various charities addressed these problems by distributing free ice to poor families for cooling milk and by providing free medical care for ill babies. In 1911 the Division of Child Hygiene established an Association of Infants' Milk Stations. Under the medical direction of Dr. Josephine Baker of the New York Department of Health, neighborhood-based milk stations provided pure milk for breastfeeding mothers or clean milk for bottle-fed infants. But even after laws were passed requiring that milk be sold in bottles, four to six bottle-fed infants died for every death of a breastfed baby.[6] Physicians advised mothers to breastfeed and warned them not to wean their babies during the summer when cow's milk stored at room temperature would spoil and give the children the dreaded "summer illness," a syndrome of diarrhea and vomiting that rapidly led to dehydration and subsequent death. Summer illness was rampant among the poor and not unknown in the middle class where mothers were constantly warned against it, sometimes in an effort to railroad them into breastfeeding.

One article published in a July 1913 edition of *The Delineator*, a stylish women's magazine sponsored by Butterick Patterns, featured a story on the value of breastfeeding illustrated by a heartbreaking photograph of a mother mourning her dead infant. The author was a doctor, Wallace B. Hamilton, who wrote with stern authority.

> We want to help save your baby. In a decade of summers, 12,468 children under five years of age died in New York City during the month of July from a single cause . . . diarrheal disease . . . And they died because their mothers did not take sufficient care in feeding and tending them. This was a preventable tragedy. The enormous Summer death rate of babies is due to a crime, the mother crime of neglect. It isn't sufficient to love your baby more than you love anything else in the world; you must safeguard his health this Summer in the most careful scientific way if you are going to keep him with you . . . Baby's food has the most to do with keeping him in good health . . . during the heat of the Summer. Proper maternal feeding is the great factor in reducing infant mortality and in bringing about baby's Summer welfare.[7]

Hamilton then went on to provide instructions for breastfeeding mothers which seemed designed to sabotage the process. Like other physicians of the day, he was schooled in schedules appropriate to the new hand or to bottle feeding and applied them without alteration to breastfeeding. "Nurse your baby at regular intervals," he charged mothers already terrified by the picture of a baby presumably dead from the mother crime of neglect. "It is not wise to allow a baby to nurse as long as he wishes. . . . Do not discontinue nursing baby, but try to detect the fault on your part. The following . . . should be looked into . . . too much food . . . too prolonged nursings, too fast nursings, irregular nursings, too frequent nursings and night nursings, too much fat in the mother's milk, milk scanty and poor in quality."[8] Clearly, hapless readers were made to feel that whatever they did in terms of breastfeeding was likely to be faulty and might well bring about the dreaded illness.

In the same issue of *The Delineator*, Nestlé's Foods printed an ad which might have looked like a reprieve to the frantic mother. Written in the same tone as Hamilton's recommendations, Nestlé offered a solution which could relieve the nursing mother of all her anxieties and inconveniences. But first the mother had to be sufficiently terrified:

> A fly in the milk one second carries death for your baby . . . Look out for flies and look out for open milk bottles . . . Look out for milk in its travels from the dairy to your baby's mouth. If you knew the cow the milk came from, who had milked the cow, if you could be with the milk from the moment it left the cow until it entered the little baby's mouth; if you could purify it and modify it, as Doctors say it should be done, you could give your baby cows' milk without fear. These things you can't do. But you can rely on Nestlé's Food that comes to you packed in an air-tight can, clean, pure, that has been watched every minute, that no hands have touched. The milk from the carefully-kept Nestlé cows, purified, modified to suit your baby's delicate digestion, that is Nestlé's Food. The addition of cold water and two minutes boiling makes it ready . . . And the coupon for twelve feedings and the book on baby's care and health. Both are free.[9]

Some sixty-five years later, Nestlé, still offering free samples to get mothers started with its product, was the major target of the largest non-union boycott against an industry in the history of the United States.[10] Grown to a huge international conglomerate, Swiss-based Nestlé S.A. had wrested 50 percent of a rich global market in infant formula that brought in two billion dollars a year, much of it from Third World nations.[11] The Infant Formula Action Coalition (INFACT), a group of concerned individuals and organizations, singled out Nestlé, not only because of its huge share of the market, but because of its particularly aggressive marketing techniques in developing countries. All formula makers, seeing a decline in sales among industrialized nations as birth rates fell or stabilized, turned their attention to new markets and used hard sell methods in advertising and promoting their products. However, Nestlé was reportedly the most adamant and least willing to listen to criticism.

Officials from UNICEF estimated that most of the annual eleven million deaths of the world's infants during the first year of life were due to malnutrition or diarrheal disease. Of these, about one million deaths could be attributed to artificial infant formulas, in a fresh outbreak of the old killer, summer illness, now referred to as "bottle baby disease." Feeding by bottle in areas where water was impure, sterilization difficult to accomplish, and refrigeration unavailable or unknown, put infants in double jeopardy. They were deprived of antibodies available in human milk which would help protect them from intestinal disease, and, at the same time, they were placed in greater risk of developing the disease through contaminated water, unsterile bottles, and bacteria in milk kept at ordinary temperatures. In the heat of tropical countries, leftover milk showed "explosive bacterial growth" within a short time.[12]

It was in just such places, INFACT charged, that Nestlé and other formula makers were responsible for the sudden and often disasterous decline in breastfeeding. In Ethiopia, Nigeria, India, and countries of Latin America, new mothers often received a free can of infant formula on discharge from the hospital. A week or so later when the can was empty, these woman often found their breasts were also empty since milk dries up without the stimulation of nursing. They also discovered that the cost of keeping their babies on formula, which had become a necessity, could consume almost the entire family income. The tragedy of summer illness or bottle baby disease deepened as mothers struggled to make formula last longer by watering it down, and their babies suffered further from malnutrition. INFACT also accused Nestlé of "employing 'milk nurses' . . . sales women in medical uniforms, to sell their products to mothers in hospitals."[13] Few women would know they were dealing with the equivalent of a "detail man" promoting drugs in physicians' offices rather than a medical professional. Officials from the World Health Organization corroborated charges about samples being given away on a grand scale. According to their figures, the average clinic in Nigeria received as many as eight thousand free cans of infant formula a year, and during the late seventies an estimated five million nursing bottles were distributed among the high-birth countries of India, Nigeria, Ethiopia, and the Philippines.[14]

No one can ascertain how much advertising and promotion were to blame for the sudden sharp conversion to bottle feeding in these and other developing countries, but it was difficult to accept the formula industries' defense that advertising had small effect and that "changing life styles" primarily accounted for the switch. The industry also argued that many Third World women, suffering from lifelong deprivation, were unable to provide sufficient milk for their babies, and that the availability of formula thus saved infants' lives. WHO clearly rejected this reasoning as a justification for sharp practice in the marketplace. Over a two-year period, two UN agencies, WHO together with UNICEF, convened delegates from governments, health institutions, and the formula industry with the aim of producing regulations on the promotion of infant formula. In May of 1981, all member nations of the UN, except one, voted to accept the resulting voluntary code. The lone negative vote was cast by the United States, in protest of what the Administration viewed as a violation of free speech and a restraint of trade. Persuaded by lobbyists who feared the code might be a precursor of regulations governing the marketing of other food products, the United States persisted in its vote even after two top officials from the Agency of International Development resigned in protest, and the nomination of an Assistant Secretary of State for Human Rights had to be withdrawn because it was discovered his tax-free research group had accepted a twenty-five thousand dollar grant from Nestlé S.A..[15]

After the WHO vote, Nestlé announced the formation of a committee to oversee its voluntary compliance with the new rules, and the attention of INFACT supporters turned to domestic concerns about infant formula. By this time it was believed in some medical circles that summer illness or bottle baby disease, while not as deadly as early in the century, was on the rise again in American ghettos and other areas where minority women were turning to bottle feeding in great numbers. Many pediatricians would agree with the figures given by Dr. Allan Cunningham of Columbia University.

"I would expect seventy-seven hospital admissions for illness in every one thousand bottle-fed infants. The comparable figure for breastfed infants is five hospital admissions."[16] Poor women, like those in the Third World, sometimes lack the facilities for proper formula preparation and milk storage, yet in the eighties these are the women most likely to put their infants on expensive formula. Nursing among Black women has declined during the past thirty years from nearly 80 percent to only 20 percent, and a significant portion of the latter figure represents educated women in the upper income brackets.[17]

Despite the setback from the controversy surrounding the WHO code and the increase of breastfeeding among middle-class mothers, selling infant formula in the United States is still good business. Annual sales amount to five hundred and fifty million dollars, shared by Abbott Laboratories (50–55 percent) Bristol Meyers (40 percent) and American Home Products (8 percent). Manufacturers have become self-appointed authorities on all aspects of infant feeding, both breast and bottle. Just as pharmaceutical companies and medical industries have come to exercise powerful influences on the nation's health care systems, formula manufacturers influence the providers of maternal child services by inundating them with information about breast feeding that is designed to sell formula.

In 1982, ICEA and other consumer organizations circulated a petition to various government agencies calling for regulations that would decrease the power of formula industries in hospitals and require clear customer information on formula packages. In support of this campaign, Angela Glover Blackwell and Lois Salisbury, two feminist lawyers, charged, "While purporting to encourage breastfeeding, the formula companies effectively sabotage the mother's confidence and access to accurate knowledge of the (lactation) process. Formula is presented as a relief from the anxiety and trouble of breastfeeding; publications of the formula industry (are) saturated with negative statements about breastfeeding."[18]

## Reign of the Experts and Loss of Maternal Confidence 1900–1960

The demands of free market enterprise were not the only reason for the turn-off of the human breast. The bias against traditional female wisdom including lore on breastfeeding had been gathering strength during an era infatuated with scientific method. As representatives of the new rationality, professionals claimed to be the ultimate authorities on child rearing including infant feeding, and modern women looked to them instead of to their female relatives for advice. Feminist historians Barbara Ehrenreich and Deirdre English have documented the enthusiasm for "scientific medicine . . . scientific housekeeping . . . (and) scientific child raising" that exploded in the twentieth century. People came to believe that " 'Experts' could solve society's problems because they were, as scientific men, by definition totally objective and above special interests of any kind. . . . Science was not just a method or a discipline, but a kind of religion."[19]

Yet scientific breastfeeding advice, as seen in Hamilton's 1913 article, was often uninformed since it was based solely on male theories instead of female experience. Two hundred years earlier, Dr. Cadogan, representing himself as a breastfeeding proponent, advised women to eliminate night feedings which was actually a prescription for decreased milk supply and the promotion of mastitis or breast infections. "Four times in four and twenty hours will be often enough to give suck. . . . By night I would not have them fed or suckled at all. It is this night feeding that makes them so over-fat and bloated."[20]

In the late nineteenth century, child rearing experts were guided by the ideas of L. Emmett Holt, pediatrician to the Rockefeller family and a member of the first board of directors of the Rockefeller Institute for Medical Research. His influential book, *The Care and Feeding of Infants*, first published in 1896, was still available in its 15th edition in 1935. Ashley Montagu, who crusaded for a return to a more benign type of infant care, (see Chapter Two) wrote of Holt's book: "During its long reign, it became the supreme household authority on the subject, the 'Dr. Spock' of its time. It was in this work that the author recommended the abolition of the cradle, no picking the baby up when it cried, feeding it by the clock, and not spoiling it with too much handling."[21] Although Holt, like Cadogan, disapproved of bottle feeding, he also gave advice that worked against the close physical relationship between mother and child that is the concomitant of nursing. Body contact was a particular target since it was believed to weaken the child, making it soft and unfit for the modern world.

The new field of twentieth-century psychology also shaped child care practices. John B. Watson, acknowledged dean of behaviorism, frowned on any parental display of affection. Children were to be treated like small adults, kept off laps and out of motherly embraces. A kiss on the forehead was allowed at night, but a manly handshake must suffice for morning. Children were to be prepared to enter an industrial world where punctuality and discipline counted, not spontaneity. Watson and other behavioral scientists advised rigid schedules that deprived babies of essential stimulation and often of normal affection. A child was a piece of clay to be molded into shape. Good habits were established by suppressing the normal impulses of childhood and forcing infants to eat, sleep, and even excrete at a specified time.

These prevailing attitudes dovetailed with institutional needs for structure and schedules. As one woman recalls from the forties, "hospital rules were well designed to kill the breastfeeding process in three days." Under medical orders, nurses sterilized the mother's nipples with alcohol, painted them with tincture of benzoin allegedly to harden them, and strapped up breasts with adhesive tape when they became engorged. "Our procedure was so regimented, baby was to be put to breast one minute the first day, three minutes the second day . . . ," a nursing sister wrote as recently as 1963.[22]

Infants placed in central nurseries were on a rigid four-hour schedule. If they grew hungry between times, they either cried themselves into exhaustion or were fed formula or sugar water by nurses. If the child was then too tired or full to suckle at the breast, the new mother had further difficulty. Almost every woman who attempted nursing for the first time during those decades remembers being told at least once by hospital staff that she was starving her child. Mothers were urged to supplement the breastfeedings with formula because their milk might be too weak (or too rich), somehow never just right as was scientific infant formula.

It was in this restrictive climate that breastfeeding in the middle class declined dramatically. Recounting breastfeeding history, Dr. Richardson wrote, "By the beginning of the century it had come to be regarded more or less as an act of God—a good trick if you could do it, but you probably couldn't."[23] Toward the end of the century, many women felt just about the same way. One of them, quoted by sociologist Linda Blachman admitted, "After I gave birth, I couldn't imagine milk coming out of my breasts any more than I could imagine milk coming out of my elbows or feet, so I didn't think it was going to."[24] This attitude cannot be totally blamed on the male experts since it was an inevitable side effect of women's struggle for freedom from old restrictions. Just as women in the twenties had campaigned for twilight sleep in labor in order to be liberated from their grandmothers' sufferings, some women fought for the bottle as a similar emblem of freedom. Thus, mothers were not eager to accept the views of the few professionals like Montagu and Dr. Margaret Ribble (*Rights of Infants*) who championed breastfeeding and old-world practices such as rocking the baby. But they did turn with relief to pediatrician Benjamin Spock who in reviving the concept of feeding a baby on demand instead of on schedule, set the stage for a return to breastfeeding later in the century (*Baby and Childcare*, Pocket Books, 1946). However, in the forties when Spock's influence was at its height, two generations of mothers had bottle-fed their infants and no longer had any living model to show them how they might do otherwise. As Raphael put it: "There (was) practically no one left who remember(ed) the old urgencies, the old tales and ways."[25]

## Niles Newton: A Scientist Attacks Medical Myths About Nursing

It was not until 1948 that a behavioral scientist focused exclusively upon the subject of breastfeeding, challenging dominant scientific attitudes with the weapons of science itself—research and statistics. Having nursed her own children, psychologist Niles Newton published ten controlled studies on human lactation between 1948 and 1958, many in collaboration with her husband, Dr. Michael Newton, who was director of the American College of Obstetricians and Gynecologists from 1966 to 1974. A longtime friend and consultant to La Leche League International, Dr. Newton belonged to the group that urged creation of ICEA. She is the mother of four children, the author or co-author of nearly sixty research papers, chapters in several books and two monographs, all on various psychophysiological aspects of women's health, a full professor of psychology at Northwestern University Medical School, a Ph.D. advisor, and a member of several editorial boards.

In 1947, she was a young mother of two daughters, working on a graduate degree at Columbia University by commuting from Philadelphia to New York City once a week. She had nursed her first baby for nearly a year and was successfully nursing the second one when she and her husband, a resident at the University of Pennsylvania Medical School, embarked on a landmark study in human lactation. Niles made a search through medical literature on the subject and found little but mythology. So she turned to veterinary journals, specifically to a dairymen's publication reporting the work of two researchers, Ely and Petersen, on the physiology of the "letdown" process in cows. Niles summarized the conclusions of the studies:

> Nerves in the teat are stimulated by sucking or milking; impulses which cause the release of the oxytocic principle of the posterior pituitary gland are carried to the central nervous system. This substance reaches the breast by the bloodstream and causes contractions of the smooth muscle surrounding the alveoli. Thus the contents of the alveoli are forced into the large ducts where they are available to the young or to the milking machine. In addition to the direct stimulus of sucking, psychic factors such as preparations for milking may initiate the reflex.[26]

The researchers had also shown that the let-down reflex was inhibited if the cows were frightened by placing cats on the backs of the animals at milking time and by popping paper bags in their ears. As might be expected, the cows gave less than their usual ration of milk.

When the Newtons set out to study the same process in nursing women, they had to face the physical and psychological barriers to experiment. "For this reason . . . we feel justified in presenting the results of well-controlled studies on one subject."[27] The subject was, in fact, Niles herself acting as observer, and seven-month-old Frances Lees Newton (Leesy) was the infant whose ability to get breastmilk from a distracted mother was the central question of the study. Since only her mother was to be disturbed, loud noises and changes in room temperature were rejected, as well as scratching cats. Also, because Niles' let-down was usually triggered by the baby's cries, the child had to be kept quiet and content each morning before the experimental feeding began when she was weighed on a highly-accurate scale and put to her mother's breast. On control days, nothing further took place except another weighing when nursing was finished.

Distraction days were a different story. Sometimes Michael Newton plunged his wife's feet in ice water, other times he pulled her big toe with increasingly painful pressure. Finally, adding humiliation and embarrassment to pain, he asked questions in math and if the answers were wrong, administered an electric shock to the nursing mother.

In addition, on each distraction day Niles received an injection either of salt water, which had no effect, or of the hormone oxytocin, which previous evidence indicated was crucial in triggering the let-down reflex in cows. That belief was borne out in the Newtons' study. Leesy received a good deal less milk on distraction mornings unless her mother was injected with oxytocin; then the amount of breast milk was almost equal to that produced on control days.

In 1948 the Newtons published the results of their experiment in *The Journal of Pediatrics:*

> Our results support the idea that Petersen's theory of the mechanism of let-down in animals holds for the lactating woman. It is interesting to speculate on the possible application of this knowledge to breast feeding in general. Many mothers are nervous about feeding their first baby; they are upset by the strange hospital surroundings; they are embarrassed at having to expose their breasts among strangers, their nipples are often sore and their breasts engorged. . . . Emotional disturbances, embarrassment, and pain inhibit let-down to the sucking baby, and thus the baby gets little milk . . . A vicious cycle is thus set up."[28]

In 1950 the Newtons published three papers on breastfeeding and three more in 1951, one under Niles' name alone, as were two the following year. In "Nipple Pain and Nipple Damage," also published in the *Journal of Pediatrics*, 1952, Niles demonstrated through a study of two hundred eighty-seven breastfeeding women that certain common hospital treatments, such as cleansing the nipples with alcohol in an attempt to make them sterile, did more harm than good. In a book that grew out of her doctoral thesis, (*Maternal Emotions*, Hoeber, 1955) she noted:

> "Unfortunately, the deep disgust many members of our contemporary society feel toward all body secretions makes rational nipple care difficult. In spite of facts to the contrary, there remains a deep unshaken emotion that a nipple, with its profusion of secretions, must be soaped or otherwise tampered with. Several other lactation rituals are similarly harmful to milk secretion—and similarly, in spite of objective evidence to the contrary, they continue to be practiced."[29]

These and other observations and research brought Niles an international reputation as an expert on human lactation. In 1963, she was invited by the World Health Organization to be a member of an international group of scientists engaged in writing a report on the physiology of lactation. As well as being the only behavioral scientist, she was the only woman on the commission.[30]

Niles became convinced that through most of human history

the process of breastfeeding had been pleasurable just as sexual intercourse was, and for the same basic reason. "The survival of the human race has long depended on the satisfactions gained from the two voluntary acts of reproduction—coitus and breast feeding. These had to be sufficiently pleasurable to ensure their frequent occurrence."[31] Between intercourse and nursing, of course, loomed childbirth, and she found a network of connection there, too. When male scientists study female sexuality, she charged, they usually focus on the one aspect that interests them most—intercourse. "Female sensuality, however, includes at least three reproductive acts that involve two persons: coitus, parturition, and lactation. It is my thesis that these three functions are closely inter-related . . . what occurs on the delivery table . . . is very pertinent to what occurs later in the marital bed; and a mother-infant relationship without enjoyable breastfeeding is in some ways similar to marriage without enjoyable sex."[32]

Newton cited evidence that oxytocin, an "orphan hormone" little explored in research, was significant in instigating these activities. She further linked all three with observational data from Kinsey's descriptions of female behavior during sexual excitement and Read's accounts of undrugged women in childbirth. There are startling correlations showing that a woman in the throes of giving birth might respond very much as if she were in the throes of orgasm. Elsewhere Newton had cited observations of a strong correlation between sexual arousal and pleasure in breastfeeding. "One of the chief difficulties," she wrote, "in viewing women's sexuality as a whole is that the taboos against some aspects of it are much greater than others. The intercourse aspect . . . is . . . freely discussed in the popular press. The experiences of childbirth and pregnancy are just beginning to be freely discussed and even photographed. . . . (However) the idea that successful breastfeeding gives sensuous pleasure is generally considered utterly unprintable!"[33] (See Elisabeth Bing's difficulty in publicizing her 1977 book on sexual intercourse for pregnant women, Chapter Two.)

Niles' confidence and ability to make fresh observations came in part, she felt, from the influence and example of a number of strong, intellectual women in her life. Her mother, Fanny Scott Rumely, who gave birth to Niles in New York in January 1923, had graduated from Smith College in 1900. While she considered mothering the most important role in her life, she also managed farms in Indiana with foresighted business acumen. Niles' father,

Edward Rumely, was a physician who practiced medicine briefly before assuming charge of the family business of manufacturing and selling farm equipment. The family lived in New York City but spent every summer in La Porte, Indiana where Dr. Rumely had founded a boys' school that emphasized manual skills as a way to increase learning ability. The Rumelys, who shared a love for children and a cheerful family life, taught their children to follow their own consciences no matter what others did. Mrs. Rumely had been raised in the Swedenborgian Church, a faith of fresh interpretations rather than orthodox views. When her children asked her about places like heaven and hell, she told them: "People probably go to hell because they feel more comfortable there."

The second strong woman in Niles' life was her nurse, Anna Becker, who helped care for her in early childhood. Anna herself had been born prematurely, and her father immediately placed her in a cigar box in the oven to keep her warm. When the tiny child miraculously survived, she became the recipient of all the love and devotion her family could give her. She bestowed that legacy willingly upon the four Rumely children, especially Niles, the youngest, who was devoted to her.

The third female influence was Millicent Carey McIntosh, head mistress of the highly regarded Brearley School in New York City where Niles enrolled at age fourteen. Along with all Brearley girls, she was expected to meet the high standards of performance set by Mrs. McIntosh who as mother of five and an efficient administrator became model for what Niles would later accomplish in her own dual career. In 1940 she graduated from Brearley and spent a year at Smith before transfering to Bryn Mawr where she majored in psychology. Impressed with the skill of good women teachers, Niles believed that women students performed better in competition with other women than they did in coeducational schools where all too often they fell into traditional roles of lower achievers.

In 1942, Niles met "the only man I didn't have to talk down to" at a Bryn Mawr dance. After a year of courtship, she and Michael Newton, an English medical student in the U.S. on a Rockefeller fellowship, were married. In 1944, Niles accompanied her husband to England where he completed medical studies. This was toward the end of World War II when there was an enormous buildup of troops and supplies in preparation for the imminent invasion of Europe. Everyone knew the invasion was coming, but no one knew where or when, and in this atmosphere of excitement and suspense,

Niles' experience seemed like a great adventure. While Michael studied for examinations at Cambridge and later worked as a casualty officer at a London hospital, Niles and another American woman ran a Red Cross canteen where G.I.s came for companionship on the eve of being shipped out to battle.

In the fall of 1944, Niles, then pregnant, left England on the Queen Elizabeth, a luxury ocean liner converted into a troop ship. In the company of British war brides and American flyers who had completed their missions, Niles traveled to New York City where in December she gave birth to a daughter, Elizabeth Willoughby, who was to be called "Willow." In 1947, the Newtons had another daughter, Frances Lees, the "Leesy" of the first breastfeeding study. In 1953, Edward Robson was born under what Niles termed "unusually fortunate circumstances," partially due to Michael Newton's position as resident in the hospital where Niles delivered. He stayed with his wife during the entire delivery which took place on a labor bed.

> Our ten-pound four-ounce baby boy arrived quickly and easily after a relaxed labor without analgesia or anesthesia. He was put to the breast while still attached to me via cord and placenta. . . . we have been together continuously except for a few brief minutes. . . . I am still amazed at the ease of my labor compared with my conventional—heavily sedated—ones, and the days I spent in the hospital getting acquainted with my son at my side will always seem to me a wonderful island of peaceful happiness in the busy stream of life.[34]

Niles insisted on rooming in with the baby. The nurses, accustomed to women with drug hangovers, worried that she'd drop her newborn on the floor, so she asked that her bed be pushed against the wall with a bedrail on the other side, enabling the baby to stay with her. "As I lay in my hospital bed and heard the screams of women in labor, and the screams of babies in the nursery, I could not help but remember that my first two children started life that way. How many of these women might like, as I did, this different way of childbearing?"[35]

Niles had met the fourth influential woman in her life a few years earlier when she and her mother took a class taught by Margaret Mead at Columbia University. Niles' knowledge about breastfeeding sparked the anthropologist's interest. As an observer of child rearing customs in exotic cultures and, like her colleague Ashley Montagu, a highly vocal critic of medical attitudes toward childbirth and breastfeeding in America, Mead found much to share with her bright young student. When Niles underwent oral exams for an interdisciplinary Ph.D. in family life education in 1952, Dr. Mead was on the examining committee. She took Niles out for a drink afterward and told her she was entering a controversial field, but the Ph.D. was something that couldn't be taken away from her.

Niles studied with Dr. Mead from 1962 to 1965, first learning how to interpret cross-cultural data in the human relations field and then collaborating with her in writing an extensive chapter: "Cultural Patterning of Perinatal Behavior," in *Childbearing: Its Social and Psychological Aspects* (Williams and Wilkins, 1967). During this period, she was exposed to Mead's theories on human relationships, including the view that the classic nuclear family was far too small and fragile for the task of bringing up children. When Mead and her third husband, the celebrated Gregory Bateson, had a daughter, they joined with another academic family in a communal setting where they shared the childrearing tasks. Nevertheless, Mead backed the fledgling childbirth movement of the fifties that developed into ICEA in 1960, supporting more conventional families who were attempting to reform maternity care. In spite of having mildly criticized childbirth education as a fad, she lent her name to the ICEA Board of Consultants and appeared to speak at its meetings. Through such associations she had met Charlotte Aiken before ICEA was founded and later made Niles aware of the Aikens' journal.

Aiken, the fifth strong influence in Niles life, was a woman of great warmth and insight whom Niles called "the grandmother of ICEA." Mrs. Aiken and her husband Gayle published a small but influential journal, *Child Family Digest*, that they had created as a memorial to one of their sons, lost in action in World War II. In an obituary following Charlotte Aiken's death in 1977, Niles wrote, "They turned their grief into public service with the hope of building a less hateful world." During a period when there was no national group encouraging childbirth reform and education, Charlotte Aiken introduced people and kept them in touch with what was going on in the movement through personal letters as well as the magazine. "The Aikens published what I wrote, which was a tremendous encouragement to a little-published author."[36]

In 1955, the Newtons moved to Jackson, Mississippi, where Michael Newton became chairman of the department of obstetrics and gynecology in the medical school of the University of Mississippi where Niles also taught. Four years later, the Newtons had another son, Warren Polk, whose entry into the world was, like his brother's, one of "unusually fortunate circumstances." During one of his American tours, Grantly Dick-Read stayed in the Newton home. Combined with friendship with the Aikens, these experiences fueled Niles' commitment to childbirth reform. She began to work with pioneer childbirth educator Mabel Fitzhugh on a shared dream of founding a national organization. When the Maternity Center Association called a meeting of those interested in reforming birth practices, Niles flew to New York City and joined the others (Hazel Corbin, Charlotte Aiken, Edith Newell, Dr. Virginia Larsen, and Mabel Fitzhugh among them) in creating the ICEA. (See Chapter Two.)

Fitzhugh, a widowed architect, had been unable to find work during the Depression. She became a physical therapist and an expert on infant posture, and from there moved into childbirth education. Learning how to prepare women for birth by observing Helen Heardman during the early days of the natural childbirth study at Grace-New Haven, Fitzhugh took it upon herself to train others in the hope that childbirth education would become universal. She held organizational meetings in her California home, and at the request of Bradley in Denver, educated Rhondda Hartman who in turn trained more teachers. When she was stumping about the country training childbirth educators, the Newtons invited her to Jackson. Subsequently, as a research associate with Michael Newton at the university for an extended period, Fitzhugh collaborated with him in designing a delivery room backrest that allowed a mother to give birth sitting upright instead of lying flat on her back.

For a number of years, Niles worked directly with Fitzhugh, Dr. Rawlins and others in strengthening the ICEA. At the medical school these activities made her controversial, and she was removed from patient contact and given an appointment in neurosurgery where animal research was underway. Undaunted, Niles decided to test her birth hypotheses on parturient mice. In collaboration with scientists Dudley Peeler and Donald Foshee, as well as Michael Newton, she observed birth outcome in groups of mice housed in various environments (covered cages, glass fish bowls), and found that mice subjected to environmental disturbances not only took significantly longer to deliver pups than control mice, but also gave birth to 54 percent more dead pups. In interpreting the data, Niles challenged American maternity practices. "Are mammals with more highly developed nervous systems (in short, human mothers) equally sensitive to perinatal environment disturbances?"[37]

In 1974, Niles confronted physicians more directly on "disturbances" they caused to humans in labor when she addressed an AMA conference titled "The National Congress On the Quality of Life." Why, she wanted to know first of all, weren't there more women speakers at a conference dealing with childhood, since women bore most of the responsibility of caring for children? "Instead we have been treated to one male speaker after another hypothesizing about what they feel childbearing women and their offspring need and want. . . . How is it possible in our society to put on a program on maternal and child health with *so little input from the mother?*" (Emphasis added.)[38] The indignation of such a query was also apparent in her further questioning of American maternity practices. Why, she asked, are expectant mothers hounded about their diets to keep their weights abnormally low? Why are rules imposed in hospitals that weaken families by separating people during childbirth? Why do physicians continue to cut episiotomies? "I do not know of a single well-controlled scientific study showing health advantages in cutting the woman's perineum as delivery approaches in normal labor. I wonder whether this custom is not part of a basic philosophic assumption that faster is always better."[39]

Newton's interest in unnecessary female surgery continued in the seventies. In a literature search on long-term effects of hysterectomy, she and a graduate student, Enid Baron, showed that the surgery often was associated with problems that might not emerge for several months, perhaps as long as a year afterward. These included higher rates of depression and psychiatric hospital admissions, as well as sex and sleep dysfunctions. Women on the average took longer to recover from hysterectomy than from other types of surgery, and many suffered from hot flashes although their ovaries had not been removed. Niles found the likely cause for this menopausal symptom in research that indicated impaired ovarian circulation from manipulations during surgery.[40]

Just as women were hesitant to complain about painful episiotomies in childbirth, they often did not question the need for a hysterectomy in later life. It was, and is, a rare woman who seeks a second opinion from one of the specialists Diane Scully called the "uterus snatchers," especially if the woman had never questioned doctors about her care in any other situation.[41] Dr. Michelle Harrison observed that compliance with medical advice is a pattern that is often set up with the first childbirth experience.[42]

For over thirty years Niles Newton has challenged practices which have tended to keep birthing and nursing women in dependent and inferior positions and has supported her argument with impeccable research. As a psychologist, she notes that much of what is considered essentially feminine in the modern world—behavior reflecting weakness, inferiority, and insecurity—came with the industrial revolution and the discounting of women's importance as childbearers and nurturers when children became economic burdens. Ironically, the biological pressures of mothering require that women be assertive, productive, and capable of concerted effort—characteristics viewed as distinctly unfeminine. After her first work produced evidence that supported women's right to nurse their infants, she found herself allied with a group that represented motherhood at its most feminine.

## La Leche: Our Lady of Bountiful Milk and Easy Delivery

Years before Niles sought out information about hysterectomy or dreamed of mice dating techniques, she had wondered when she nursed Willow why she, as an enlightened and educated mother, should worry so much about such a simple process. In 1953, she wrote in the *Child Family Digest:* "Helping mothers breastfeed today is . . . more difficult than it was a hundred years ago in spite of the fact that we know more physiology. . . . A hundred years ago a girl grew up seeing her mother, her aunts, and her older sister breastfeeding. . . . Almost everyone a girl met regarded breastfeeding as one of the natural rhythms of life that continued for at least a year with each baby."[43]

"The problem now," she explained in a 1960 issue of the *Digest,* "is not breastfeeding knowledge, but the application of what we already know. That is why when I heard about the work of the League from Charlotte Aiken, I flew up to Chicago (in 1956) with my own breastfed baby to see what they were doing. . . . I attended a meeting of the Franklin Park group. . . . Chairs were arranged in a big circle . . . nine babies snuggling in their mothers' arms. . . . During the course of the evening most were unobtrusively nursed. Thus the mothers attending the meeting had a little practical demonstration of what their great grandmothers saw all around them throughout their growing up years."[44]

The founders describe the origin of their remarkable organization in *La Leche League Love Story:* "In 1956 seven women joined together in a movement that was to change the face of motherhood in America."[45] Bound by a common belief in the value of family life and the role of lactation in preserving it, the women quietly worked to "demedicalize breastfeeding," as Barbara Katz Rothman described it a quarter of a century later.[46] In spite of the fact that it was an era in which "belief in the near miraculous powers of doctors and their medicines was at an all-time high," the League began organizing groups of women in support of breastfeeding, often in direct opposition to medical advice.[47]

"It just didn't seem fair," said Marian Tompson, "that mothers who bottle feed . . . were given all sorts of help . . . but . . . when a mother was breastfeeding, the only advice she was given was to give the baby cow's milk."[48] Marian had a friend, Mary White, wife of a family doctor, Gregory White, who favored natural birth and breastfeeding, too. The idea of the League germinated at a picnic the two women attended in midsummer of 1956. Mary White was then nursing her sixth baby, and Marian who had struggled unsuccessfully to nurse her first three babies but finally succeeded with the fourth, encouraged by Dr. White, had been wondering how she might help other women.

Now, as the two friends sat chatting under a tree while Mary White fed her infant, they thought they had the answer — a combination of what both of them had learned from experience and encouragement of the sort Dr. White had so freely given. Why not create a group to offer that aid to other women in the community? Within a few days they had asked five others to join them, women they knew through their parish church or from Dr. White's practice: Edwina Froehlich, Viola Lennon, Betty Wagner, Mary Ann Kerwin, and Mary Ann Cahill, all mothers of several children. These became the seven founding mothers and remained at the heart of the organization throughout its phenomenal growth.

Their plan was simply to offer encouragement and information to their friends and neighbors through informal classes and an instruction pamphlet. But this plan rapidly expanded as groups grew large, split off, and new groups sprouted elsewhere. Soon the League leaders were innundated with frantic telephone calls and letters from mothers all over the country, asking for help in breastfeeding. Finding that early feeding of solid foods was affecting women's ability to continue breastfeeding, they studied the nutritional needs of mother and infant and suggested that the early introduction of solid foods was not necessary. This theory ran counter to prevailing medical opinion and social fashion in a time when women vied with each other on how early they could get a spoonful of cereal down the baby.

Doctors objected to the League's stand, but the leaders held fast because they realized women who had nursed and subsequently weaned infants knew more about the subject than any man, regardless of his medical education. In fact, they decided, many of the questions about nursing were not medical concerns at all, but those of mothering. This was an amazing stance for such a group of women, none feminist by any standard nor interested in women gaining power and authority in spheres beyond the family. But what they knew, they knew, and stuck to with passionate intensity. Gregory White notes in *Love Story* that there were other groups for nursing mothers, but they had all been run by medical professionals teaching women rather than women helping one another. As a mother wrote in the *La Leche League News:* "My doctor has never nursed a baby. He knows how to put in stitches, this sort of thing. Sally Jones has nursed three babies . . . Darlene Smith has nursed four. . . . That is why I call them instead of my doctor."[49]

Single-minded devotion to one cause has been the hallmark of the League in its quarter century of existence. Its leaders have always considered the League a one-issue organization, focused only on support for breastfeeding and not involved in political questions that might arise from that support. In an early edition of the *News*, Betty Wagner defined the League by a process of elimination. "We are not teaching 'cancer' prevention; we are not teaching 'nutrition'; we are not teaching 'family planning'; we are teaching mothering through breastfeeding."[50]

The League held fast to this policy when it was informally invited by the medical profession to become its subsidiary in the milk bank business. Nutritionist Alan Berg's description of mother's milk as "a wasted natural resource," in 1976,[51] had been picked up by the media, instigating what Edwina Froelich termed "a rediscovery of human milk by the scientific community (who began) following up studies of Derrick B. Jeliffe, Paul Gyorky, and Niles Newton."[52]

Doctors, belatedly acknowledging the protective value of human milk, began to prescribe it for sick and premature infants, and local League groups were asked to contribute milk for infants in neonatal nurseries. "We began to have several requests for milk a week. It taxed our volunteers. I was not asked to deliver the milk (at my own expense and time). I was told to get it to the unit right away or a baby would die. I was also told we could not contact the mother and the implication was that somehow, I, not she, was responsible for this life or death situation," reported a League Leader in 1978.[53] Committed fiercely to the volunteer ethic of service without pay, League leaders did not complain that women were never paid for the milk (the going price from milk banks was $1.25 an ounce in the early eighties), whereas men were routinely paid for their semen samples. A milk bank representative glibly explained this discrepancy. Women, he said, could easily dilute their milk to make more money.[54] In 1977 the League issued an information sheet clarifying its position: "We do not function as a milk bank . . . we cannot offer to supply breast milk for a longer period of time (than three weeks). That period should be enough . . . to get started on re-lactation or for you to find another source of milk."[55]

On this question as on others, the League held fast to its independence and insistence that in this field women, not professionals, were the experts. Barbara Katz Rothman noted that of all the groups centering on reforming childbirth and mother-infant care, the League alone remained firmly outside the sphere of professional control and consistently refused to be co-opted by the medical establishment. She honored the League for having presented a woman-centered model of mothering, one in which the mother is the expert. "The League is certainly not 'feminist'. . . . women are, in their view, bound totally to home and child, and mothering is the only role they seem to see for a woman. On the other hand, within that domain she is in control and her judgement is valued."[56]

This view and the League's wholehearted commitment to breasts as the source of not only nourishment but nurturing (The motto was, 'Good mothering through breastfeeding.') exposed certain fundamental ambiguities in American culture. Foremost among these was the contrast between the function of breasts as milk producers and as sexual ornaments for the pleasure of males.

## Breastfeeding and Sex

By the 1950s a combination of factors had brought breastfeeding, at least in public, to such disfavor it was thought of as only slightly less impolite than other excreting activities, a phenomenon that Niles Newton remarked upon. On the one hand, breasts molded by the brassiere to fit the fashion for separation and well-defined points, breasts of the sort the entertainer Cher described as "standing at attention,"[57] and breasts whose confinement in tight bodices produced deep, heaving cleavage were fair game for symbolizing sexuality on covers of books, in movies and advertisement, and on the pinup posters that decorated the lockers of American G.I.s all over the world. Since the genital area was still almost taboo, even in sex magazines, the breasts seemed to have been made a substitute. In fact, from casual observation, the bosom might have appeared as the actual site of sexual gratification.

At the same time, extreme prudery surrounded any mention of the functioning breast (which, of course, had to be attached to the nursing mother), and deviance from the code forbidding public breastfeeding was associated with lower-class ignorance. One woman, a nursing mother in the fifties, said that the only place she could nurse in a restaurant was while perched on a toilet seat in the restroom.

American culture was still well in the grip of such restrictive attitudes when LLLI held its first convention in 1964. Interestingly enough, the delegates met in a hotel near Chicago Playboy Club, a juxtaposition which Dr. Robert Mendelsohn was quick to note:

> It seems to me that some of the most basic conflicts in our society are dramatically exemplified by the activities and attitudes in these two places. . . . The physical proximity of these two groups is in dramatic contrast to their emotional and psychological distance. Both have certain superficial similarities. In both breasts are emphasized, on the one hand for strictly ornamental purposes and in a suggestive fashion, on the other hand for certain functions. . . . What are breasts for?[58]

Had Niles Newton been asked to comment, she might have said that a woman's breasts cannot be viewed as belonging in one sphere or the other, but as part of her sexual being with the capacity to respond to her infant as well as her lover. She might have added that the survival of the human race had depended for millenia on the pleasure to be gained from nursing, as well as that from intercourse. Although the League was not concerned with the erotic capacities of breasts, they did see their value as more than providing nourishment. League principles clustered around a belief that good mothering grew out of an attachment between mother and infant that occurred most naturally in breastfeeding. Their remarkable success has been in the transformation of societal attitudes within a generation, so that today breastfeeding infants is viewed among the educated middle class as the most desirable form of feeding. However, this tolerance is limited to nursing babies for about nine months to a year at most. Any mother who continues to nurse an older child is sure to be regarded with a certain amount of horror and the barely concealed judgment that something other than nourishing is going on.

According to Jimmy Lynn Avery, editor of the now-defunct journal *Abreast of the Times*, the most common medical argument against breastfeeding after the child's first year is based on the fear that "the mother does it for her own emotional (i.e. sexual) needs."[59] Thus, in the present day, despite the sexual revolution, pleasure in breastfeeding beyond a time when it can comfortably be considered vital to the child's food needs is still taboo. All along, of course, some women doggedly continued to nurse toddlers, usually half in secret, terming themselves as Avery did, "closet nursers."

Discovering that the medical rule on weaning babies at nine months was not based on any solid evidence, the League leaders decided once again they were asking the wrong people for guidance. "Since it wasn't a medical question, their (the doctors') medical education was no help. That was why no good answer could be found in the medical books. We decided that it would be much more likely to be *a woman, a mother*, who would know."[60]

However, many women didn't know or found themselves shaken in their own judgment by the reaction of others, as happened to a young mother in a *Ms* story, "Viva's Breastfeeding Caper" published in 1975. Viva, a closet nurser, was confronted by a friend who was "horrified to find Emma (Viva's daughter) still sucking tit at fifteen and a half months." Persuaded to wean the baby immediately, Viva sought medical help. The first doctor suggested that she rub the baby's back instead of nursing her. The second advised an abrupt halt: "Cold turkey, that's the only way to do it." Unable to endure the resulting pain, Viva tried a third doctor, the baby's pediatrician. Appalled by the "obscene" spectacle of a sixteen month old fondling her mother's nipples right in front of him, he prescribed a breast pump. Viva described the aftermath:

> The next day was, again, sheer hell. . . . Big drops of milk were seeping out and soaking my T-shirt. . . . Emma looked longingly at the breast nearest her head and burst into tears. There seemed to be no reason at all to wean her. . . . What if I never had another child and would never

again experience a baby sucking milk at my breast? . . . Knowing . . . that I was more concerned about the experience ending for me than for the baby, I felt guilty and selfish on top of everything else.[61]

"Never have I been so upset by any article," wrote one reader. "Viva's story has about it such a frivolous attitude (that it) could dissuade a young mother from nursing by making breastfeeding sound like an orgy." Another wrote, "The story of Viva's breastfeeding caper made my day. My daughter of four . . . a beautiful, pink, plucky child, still climbs into our bed every morning to nurse." Yet another: "I am suppressing a desire to scream, to strangle about 90 percent of the country's doctors, and tell Viva what an idiot she was to listen to people telling her to wean her child."[62]

## Breastfeeding and Maternal Guilt

If women are made to feel guilty because they keep the baby at the breast too long, they are equally guilt-stricken over failures to nurse long enough or to nurse at all, particularly as breast milk has come to be recommended among childbirth educators as best for the baby. Dr. Judith Lumley points out that lactation is "particularly liable to be seen as a preventive and a remedy for individual and social evils. . . . No wonder that when breastfeeding goes wrong women feel that more is at stake than nutrition."[63]

In 1981, health educator Linda Blachman lashed out at the League and breastfeeding authors Dana Raphael and Karen Pryor for misleading women on the experience of motherhood by romanticizing breastfeeding. "Romanticism is the solution often chosen by women to avoid fear of facing our demons, to avoid the process of 'dancing in the dark.' "[64] Her two-part essay "Dancing in the Dark" is a rare exploration of the hidden side of maternity: those fears, furies and resentments that are forbidden mention in our culture and, therefore, assumed not to exist, except perhaps among the poor and ignorant. All-giving mother love is assumed to be automatic and instinctual, and the darker aspects of maternity are acknowledged neither among the earnest proponents of breastfeeding nor among those in favor of formula feeding, nor by any of the child-care experts, unless as a prelude to the accusation of child abuse. Blachman connected her criticism of undoubted League bias on the issue with her own bitter experience in weaning a four-month-old infant 'cold turkey.' She suffered not only physical pain but the emotional pain of listening to her daughter cry for twenty-four hours before the baby gave in and accepted a bottle. Nevertheless, her essays provide needed perspective on the subject of maternal guilt over breastfeeding.

Other sources of guilt lie in wait for the new mother, of course. One of these is embedded in the medical model of pregnancy which sees the needs of the mother as different from those of her fetus and infant. When pregnancy and delivery are treated as illness, Barbara Katz Rothman writes, the mother, presumably having suffered an ordeal, needs time away from her newborn so that she may recuperate. "Infants are perceived as 'demanding' . . . the infants's 'demands' are then counter to the mother's 'need for rest.' "[65]

This paradox permeates contemporary pediatric literature which on one hand subscribes to the bonding theories of Reva Rubin and Marshall Klaus (see Chapter Five) and on the other advises women to decrease contact with their infants. In a 1982 article, "The Management of Night Waking In Older Infants," pediatric nurse practitioner Janet B. Younger discusses the very real conflict between parental and infant needs when children wake frequently during the night, and prescribes a cure which sounds very like the rules of L. Emmett Holt. "The treatment is to completely stop going to the child in the middle of the night . . . be prepared for the baby's crying to range from one hour to the better part of the night. . . . Some . . . think this type of treatment is too harsh. I have never had a parent report any harmful effects."[66] In contrast, ASPO pioneer Elly Rakowitz advises the mother troubled by night waking to "consider taking the baby into bed with you. . . . Simply attach baby to nipple and go back to sleep."[67]

As tempting and natural as such advice would seem, it is a rare young mother who has the courage to follow it. First there is the child experts' warning that taking baby into a grown-up bed sows the seeds of future sexual problems. A second more immediate fear, encouraged by hospital nurses and infant-care manuals, is that the mother will roll over in her sleep and smother the baby, a tragedy that rarely if ever takes place. In fact, there is evidence that the old tales about such deaths were actually due to an occasional accident of drunkenness or, more often, served as explanations covering deliberate infanticide.

As part of their aim to alter cultural views of good child care, the League has reassured mothers that responding to their babies' cries was the proper thing to do. The League is frequently criticized for this stand, just as it is accused of making mothers feel guilty if they don't succeed in breastfeeding. Some physicians give this reason for refusing to refer their patients to the League. During a symposium on Counseling Approaches to the Breastfeeding Mother in 1980, a doctor acknowledged, "One of the things that bothered them (doctors) is the La Leche dictum that if you don't breastfeed, you have failed. . . . Hence these physicians were a little reluctant to have La Leche League involved."[68]

A member of the professional panel, Niles Newton responded: "I do not believe that La Leche League intends to make mothers feel guilty. I believe that the reason the League is unpopular among some professionals is that it's a self-help group that is tremendously successful. Professionals are always up against it when the consumer has something good going." Another doctor added: "It is threatening for a professional person to realize that a lay person knows more about something than he does."[69]

## Breastfeeding and Working Mothers

The question of whether the League is guilty of producing guilt over a failure in breastfeeding is unresolved and perhaps not even relevant. However, there is clearly a long-standing disagreement about working mothers, with the League firmly committed to a traditional ideal of every mother married to a man who is able to fully support his family while his wife stays at home with the children. In fighting for the traditional family, the League and, particularly, the founding mothers have consistently opposed a national system of day care and have frowned on the use of baby sitters during infancy, despite the increasing numbers of working mothers.

By the early eighties, economic pressures as well as changing roles of women had brought six million mothers of pre-school children into the job market, and records showed that one quarter of all women who gave birth would be at work four months later. Only one in five American families could afford to live on one salary, and one in three women who divorced had to return to work immediately. Sociologist Joseph McFalls predicted in 1982 that in the future, "only wealthy women will be able to eschew the then almost universal norm of female employment by opting for the relatively luxurious life style of being solely a wife and mother."[70]

During a homebirth conference in 1979, three employed mothers, Drs. Merilyn Solomon, Victoria Shauf, and Anne Seiden, pointed out the opposing forces that made life difficult for working mothers, one pushing women toward increasing employment and the other pulling toward a return to breastfeeding and natural mothering. They criticized the government for having done so little to make these trends compatible, while other nations have found means to sponsor child care services at the sites of employment. The women further criticized a League booklet on breastfeeding and working, charging it "may induce guilt by offering advice to the working mother only as the second best solution. The unfortunate result for many working women has been to deny themselves both the real advantages of breastfeeding and the practical assistance of a support group."[71]

Some League members have offered support to working mothers despite national policy. In 1965, Lynn Moen, the first League leader in the state of Washington and a working mother who ran the ICEA Supply Center for fifteen years, affirmed her belief that employed mothers can breastfeed. She noted that Niles Newton had supported the possibility of working while nursing, citing the case of a woman doctor who had nursed five babies, feeding them before she left in the morning and on her return in the evening, and of a local League member who worked as a musician with the Seattle symphony and reported that several of her colleagues were nursing mothers. During intermissions, "all would make a dash for the ladies' room to express some milk." Lynn also knew a woman attorney who had breastfed each of her three children for nearly a year.[72]

The League leaders responded that it's all very well to talk about doctors and lawyers and other professionals who often have the freedom to make their own schedules and the money to hire household help. But for women in ordinary white and blue collar jobs who make up four-fifths of the entire female working force, the luxury of such choices doesn't exist. An ICEA nursing mothers' counselor employed part-time added, "Choice is not always part of returning to work; it is the need for money. There is, however, an unrealistic expectation on the part of educated women who may have some choice in the matter. They want to do it all: have a splendid career, beautiful children, and a husband doing his fair share of housework and child care. For a few this is possible; (but) most of the women become disillusioned from sheer fatigue."[73]

Although various solutions have been recommended in addition to onsite day care, including flexible working hours and work that can be done at home, the League has been slow to alter its stand. In 1982, however, plans were made to publish two books for working mothers who breastfeed, as a means of revising policy. The founders apparently have difficulty recognizing that they themselves are prime examples of working mothers successfully operating at home. While unpaid at the beginning of their careers, each one put in as much time as if fully employed, and present-day leaders still follow that model, enduring a demanding schedule that consists of telephone crisis counseling and home meetings which they direct while juggling a baby on their hips.

## Radicals Rise from the Ranks of the LLLI

As the League founders and original leaders struggled to maintain the traditional family in the midst of a changing world, an atmosphere that encouraged questioning and rejecting establishment rules percolated through the ranks, producing some members who pushed for more radical reforms than the League thought wise. In 1976 founder Mary White wrote in *Leaven*, the League's professional newsletter,: "We want to remind our leaders in no case should a . . . leader encourage a home birth in which no medical attendance is planned."[74] *The News* warned the membership a month later that "home births were not practical for everyone."[75]

However, hundreds of League followers and some leaders who could not find doctors willing to attend them in their homes ignored this advice and chose the services of lay midwives to avoid the high-tech hospital birth of the seventies. One of them was Lee Stewart of Chapel Hill, North Carolina, whose husband "caught" each of their five children in home births. Like Lester and Bill Hazell, the Stewarts were members of the educated middle class. Lee was a League leader and with her husband, David, a seismologist with a doctorate in mathematics, served as Southern regional director for the ICEA. For two years, Dave was a member of the ICEA Subcommittee on Home Birth with Lester Hazell and Margot Edwards. Feeling that little was being accomplished, he and Lee founded the National Association of Parents and Professionals for Safe Alternatives in Childbirth (NAPSAC), in 1975, which rapidly replaced followers of the Bradley method as the advance guard of childbirth reform.

NAPSAC attracted a fiercely partisan and sometimes uneasy mixture of feminists determined to wrest from the male establishment women's rights to control their own reproduction, and traditionalists committed to preserving the integrity of the old self-reliant, self-contained American family. Lee Stewart, president of the new group, quoted Doris Haire in an introduction to one of a series of NAPSAC books: "It is a comment on our times that we who want childbirth to again become an intimate family affair are considered radicals."[76]

NAPSAC rallied support when Gregory White and his son William, also an M.D., had their hospital privileges revoked abruptly in December of 1981. Acknowledged authorities on home birth, their low-key activities had eventually provoked colleagues into retaliation. While the Whites were cleared of charges in 1982, their case represented one of many harassments against health care providers who questioned the rule that all babies must be born in hospitals. Responding to the nationwide increase in persecution and prosecution of alternative providers, in most cases lay midwives, NAPSAC established a legal arm, the Alternative Birth Crisis Coalition (ABCC).

A 1982 issue of *Mother Earth News* described an ABCC convention that year as a "grim assemblage of physicians, midwives, nursing mothers, and other parents gathered in Washington D.C. . . . to protect the rights of those who want to have, or participate, in home births. . . . Yet the final speaker, the executive director of ABCC, managed both to be realistic about the battle ahead and to speak with joy."[77]

That speaker was Marian Tompson, who twenty-five years earlier had accepted the presidency of the League because she thought it probably wouldn't be difficult, although she was "a rather quiet and shy person . . . a homebody who had no car to use during the day . . . alone in my neighborhood in my philosophy of child rearing, but never . . . compelled to convert anyone to my way of thinking."[78] A quarter of a century later, after the League had grown from that first meeting with six friends to La Leche League International (LLLI) with 10,000 chapters in forty-three countries, Marian Tompson was on the front line of yet another struggle, this time for people's rights to choose the place of birth. The journalist lauded her staying power. "Marian Tompson's most striking quality is her remarkable purity of spirit. Whereas many home birth supporters have understandably become embittered . . . Marian remains clear and compassionate."[79]

All childbirth reformers had good reason for both bitterness and pessimism as the decade opened. The undoubted success of the

League in rescuing breastfeeding from a dying art was offset by a new burst of medical technology which threatened nearly all the advances made by reformers in the past decade. Questions about how this challenge should be met were more complex and not so readily answered, as Elisabeth Bing had foreseen.

> How can we support this machine age without losing our . . . humanity? . . . This is a very real question . . . for all of us who fought for the participation of the parents in giving birth to their child. . . . Then, the main part of the fight was only against over-dosages of medication, almost an easy fight in retrospect. . . . The lines of battle are . . . more intricate today. Are safety and electronics synonymous?[80]

# FOUR

# Saga of Obstetrical Technology

Heralding the arrival of a new wave of obstetrical technology, in November 1976, *Newsweek* announced, "Dramatic advances have revolutionized the process of birth . . . fetal monitors prevent cases of brain damage . . . newborn intensive care units will halve the rate of U.S. infant mortality . . . high frequency sound waves are being used as a diagnostic tool during pregnancy." One physician was quoted as saying that stopping and starting labor with drugs would benefit normal pregnancies.[1] As the new machines transformed hundreds of simple labor rooms into high-risk centers, obstetricians felt an enormous excitement over what promised to be an intriguing phase of research combined with treatment that would lower the still embarrassingly high perinatal mortality rate of twenty deaths per thousand live births.

During this period, the image of childbirth fluctuated between the dangerous illness concept promoted by DeLee earlier in the century and the natural or normal model upheld by the childbirth reformists. A *McCall's* survey in 1976 showed that obstetricians were partial to the illness model. While three-quarters were willing to accept prepared parents as patients, comments made in the margins of the *McCall's* questionaire indicated an underlying doubt that women might actively participate in childbirth. "Only ten percent can do it," was one response, and another asserted that women took classes because of "personal insecurities." Dr. John Franklin, one of the founders of Booth Maternity Hospital in Philadelphia, told the *McCall's* interviewer: "Every doctor enjoys his interventions. That's what his skill and training are for. Some think that nature is in constant need of improvement, and others that nature cannot be trusted. But one intervention leads to another and then the doctor is kept busy seeking remedies for his own actions."[2]

The history of obstetrics is the history of its tools and interventions. Indeed, there are grounds for the belief that without technology, the specialty, almost totally a male province, might never have come into existence at all. Developments made to assist a woman with a difficult birth have been, with rare exceptions, the property of male accoucheurs who often used their lifesaving tools to turn a trade into a profession and advance themselves. In a typical instance, after Ambroise Paré, surgeon to the king of France, re-introduced the technique of version and extraction in the 1500s, there was an immediate increase in the numbers of men entering what would become the field of obstetrics.[3] As taught by Paré, internal version was used in cases where a child lay sideways in the uterus and could not be born. The attendant inserted a hand into the uterus, grasped the child by its feet, turned it and then pulled it out still holding the feet, in fortunate cases, saving its life. There was conflicting evidence concerning whether female midwives used version. One historian claimed the technique was used equally by male and female birth attendants. Another said that women did not have the requisite strength and intellect, and, thus the maneuver remained the domain of men "with minds more alert than women's."[4]

If version served to advance male midwives professionally, the invention of obstetric forceps, considered one of the greatest instruments of all times, hugely expanded the opportunities for their intervention. Like version, forceps were used for mechanical obstructions in childbirth, particularly when a child was caught in the womb because its head was too large to pass through the mother's pelvis. Invented by Peter Chamberlen in 1588 and kept a family secret for over a century, the new extractors brought fame and fortune to the Chamberlens. The original Chamberlen, a barber surgeon transplanted from France to England, was something of a progressive. In the words of an historian, he was "one of the great eccentrics of his time. . . . He frequently proposed to incorporate the midwives (whom he'd watched deliver with spoons and thus presumably gotten the idea of forceps) . . . (He) wished to reconcile all the Churches (and) . . . anticipated motor-cars."[5] But the tactics used by the Chamberlens to keep others from learning their life saving secret were of such bizarre proportions—ringing bells to confuse would-be observers, blindfolding family members in the birth room, and delivering under a sheet—that they blotted the reputation of the entire family.[6]

Crude and admittedly dangerous as they were, internal version and obstetric forceps represented an immense improvement over earlier solutions to mechanical obstruction in birth. These had included operating upon the mother once she died in hope of removing a living child (or at least baptizing it, whatever its condition) or crushing the child's head with cranioblasts or hooks in order to pull it out piecemeal. Of these dreadful options, Hugo Chamberlen, grandson of Peter, wrote in 1672 in a foreword to the English translation of Francis Mariceau's obstetrical text: "My father, my brother, and myself . . . (though none else in Europe as I know) have, by God's blessing and our own industry, attained to and long practiced a way to deliver women, in this case, (that is, difficult labors) without any prejudice to them or their infant . . . though all others must and do, endanger, if not destroy, one or both using hooks."[7]

When the secret of the forceps construction came out about 1720, their use exploded, allowing little time for refinement of technique. Male midwives applied the new tools so frequently that physicians themselves objected, including one William Hunter who said bitterly that "nature had apparently abandoned her work of procreation and left it to forceps." Although he himself carried a pair, he seldom used them, saying, "the better the midwife, the thicker the rust."[8]

Later in the century, there was inevitable reaction against the instruments because of frequent forceps-related injuries to both infant and mother (in the latter, lacerations and the more serious fistulas caused by tears between the vagina and bladder or rectum). This brought about a brief return to nonintervention which ended abruptly after a beloved young English princess died in childbirth in 1817 while Sir Richard Croft, accoucheur to the royal family, stood by doing nothing during a fifty-two hour labor. When the infant, who would have been heir to the throne, was born dead and the mother, Princess Charlotte, died six hours later,

Croft shot himself as the only way out of professional disgrace.[9]

When forceps and version were brought to America by doctors who had studied abroad, their use was identified with progress. As in Europe, the interventions were sometimes applied inappropriately. In the treatment of placenta previa, for example, internal version which involved pulling the leg of the fetus down into the vagina might be used in an attempt to stop hemorrhage. The maneuver was also used in cases of eclampsia and for stalled labors of all types. Toward the end of the nineteenth century, external version by manipulating the unborn infant through force of hands on the woman's abdomen began to be preferred.

Debates in medical literature of the nineteenth century over the use and abuse of both version and forceps raised ethical questions about the advance of medical science and its impact upon human welfare. Perhaps more than any other single issue, the controversy reflected the ebb and flow of enthusiasm for obstetrical technology with physicians sharply divided on whether childbirth should be left to nature or managed with interventions. As one example, Dr. Chandler R. Gilman, representing the conservative side, advised medical students at the New York College of Physicians and Surgeons from 1841 to 1865 that "Dame Nature is the best midwife in the world. . . . Meddlesome midwifery is frought with evil. . . . The less done generally the better."[10]

Advocates of both interventionist and conservative approaches often urged their theories at meetings of the American Gynecological Society. In 1878, Dr. Thomas Addis Emmet, a follower of the famed gynecological pioneer, J. Marian Sims, proposed that forceps be used not only more frequently but earlier in labor because of the alleged dangers of spontaneous delivery. "One who was familiar with the mechanism of labor, but wanting in practical experience, could do less damage in the application of a pair of forceps, than if he left the delivery, in such a case, to the efforts of nature."[11]

In 1881, Dr. Albert Smith objected to the promotion of axis-traction forceps popularized in 1877 for high forceps delivery, not on the basis of their potential for damage, but because the more complicated instruments might deter doctors from using forceps at all. A man who regarded the instruments as the way of eliminating suffering in all labors, Smith said, "The forceps operation . . . should not be looked upon as a great, magnificent operation, to be performed only by the expert . . . but as the means of relief to be given to every woman in suffering with whom the life of her child, or her own subsequent convalescence . . . may be risked by unnecessary delay."[12]

At the Fourth Annual Meeting, in 1879, Dr. Isaac Taylor presented a paper titled "The Early Application of the Forceps in the First Stage of Natural Labor," declaring he hadn't seen "any bad results in the application of forceps where the os uteri was dilated to the size of a fivecent piece or seven-eighths of an inch."[13] (One of the required conditions before a forceps delivery may be performed today is full dilation of the cervix.) At the same meeting, the president of the Society, T. Gaillard Thomas, made what might be regarded as a definitive statement of the conservative position when he criticized trachelorrhaphy (cervical repair). "No one familiar with . . . trachelorrhaphy can doubt the beneficent results of that excellent conservative procedure and yet even that seems destined to do a certain amount of evil before it stands upon reasonable middle ground. . . . If every man of the future is to inflict upon her who bears him, of necessity, a surgical operation, then will a new field of industry have opened."[14]

Actually, the new field of industry in gynecological surgery was already well-established and had been since J. Marion Sims, an Alabama doctor, developed sutures for the repair of vesico-vaginal fistulas, terrible injuries of childbirth often caused by over zealous use of forceps. Women thus torn were rendered not only invalids for life but unfit for human company due to the odors of constant seepage. Sims, who perfected surgical techniques by operating on female slaves, was viewed as a savior.

He moved on from essential repair to a number of other surgical procedures on female organs and opened his own hospital for these treatments in New York City in 1855. Surgeons who followed this "Architect of the Vagina," made further explorations; indeed, some doctors grew so enthusiastic over the possibilities, they advocated leaving very little of the female condition to nature. Sharing a national enthusiasm for expansion, in which the task was to conquer rather than protect nature, they injected the female tract with caustics, curreted the uterus, and inserted metal pessaries to hold the uterus in a "better" position. The cervix was incised for "mechanical" menstruation and, in labor, forced open with fingers, "tents," and dilators.[15] In cases where the membranes ruptured early, physicians sometimes douched the woman to lubricate the birth canal for the subsequent version and extraction. During one decade of "ovarian mayhem," surgeons removed the female ovaries for a host of alleged "nervous" and functional disorders that included sexual problems, and performed female circumcision and clitoridectomy as cures for unacceptable behavior.[16]

After the turn of the century, women were no longer subjected to terrible sexual surgeries, but American medical men wielded forceps more frequently than doctors in other countries, and version was still employed, partly out of desperation because the cesarean section remained a life-threatening surgery and partly from habit. In DeLee's view in 1916, both version and high forceps operations had little to recommend them, the former being "often difficult and laborious . . . The child is often lost by the untimely detachment of the placenta, and the uterus is sometimes ruptured in the effort to turn the child . . . The high forceps operation . . . is very bloody, and nearly always the mother's tissues suffer severe injury."[17]

Version gradually fell into disrepute in the twentieth century, although the external form and the Wright maneuver (using a combination of external and internal versions) were occasionally performed. One hold-out enthusiast for the internal procedure, Irving White Potter (*The Place of Version in Obstetrics*, 1922), advised its routine use for shortening second-stage labor. Potter, who used version in 90 percent of all his obstetrical cases, frequently demonstrated his technique on deeply-anesthetized women.[18]

In 1933, the Children's Bureau made an analysis of 7,537 maternal deaths in fifteen states and found that the women had died from three causes: living in poverty circumstances, sepsis from abortion, and the effects of hasty, ill-judged operative procedures by doctors. "Many were operated upon after very little or no labor. The number of cases in which manual dilation of the cervix, forceps or version and manual removal of the placenta occurred . . . was deplorably large. From this, it was evident that accouchment force was resorted to many times and accouchment force is not recognized as good obstetrics today."[19]

The Bureau's concept of good obstetrics may not have corresponded with currently acceptable medical practice, especially the common interferences termed "accouchement force." While the influential DeLee deplored the abuse of version and high forceps, he thought all women should be delivered with low forceps. After his success in the twenties in convincing his fellow obstetricians that "parturition, viewed with modern eyes, is no longer a normal function," his prophylactic operation using low forceps just prior to the crowning of the head became the accepted protocol in American delivery rooms.[20] Country doctors who would not use the instruments were regarded as hopelessly backward and, in time, were succeeded by younger doctors whose training had persuaded them their moral duty lay in using forceps in the service of womankind.

The popularity of forceps continued through the next decade. By 1968, the rate was frequent but variable, ranging from 10 to 90 percent depending on the hospital under survey, and medical regulation boards seldom questioned their use, concentrating instead on frequency of cesarean section where a rate over 3 percent was a signal for investigation.[21] One best-selling guide for pregnant women, revised and reissued in 1973, assured its readers: "Many babies these days are delivered by forceps. . . . Forceps, never applied without some form of anesthesia, . . . are no longer used to deliver babies from high in the birth canal. They are used only to bring the baby's head over the mother's perineum. . . . It often permits the obstetrician to shorten the second stage of labor by as much as an hour or more, thereby sparing the mother that much more pain and preventing a number of spontaneous accidents which might occur at this crucial stage."[22]

The triumph of the childbirth reformists, although they are seldom given credit for it, lay in overturning medical devotion to the prophylactic forceps operation. Success came in part from efforts by women like Hazel Corbin, Niles Newton, Elisabeth Bing, Margaret Gamper, Lester Hazell and Helen Wessel supported by a handful of unconventional physicians—Irwin Chabon, Harlan Ellis, Murray Enkin, and John Miller, in addition to those already mentioned.[23] They succeeded in some transformation of the American way of birth, in part because cultural confrontations of the sixties aided their cause. Rebellion against the old forms and old guard by students, racial minorities, farm workers, and women whipped up winds of change everywhere, and people began to openly question the wisdom of established authority, including the nearly sacred preserve of medicine. Women, searching for liberation, demanded more responsibility for their own health and a larger share in medical decisions. Natural childbirth, or Lamaze, as it came to be termed, was seen as an extension of this philosophy. In addition, the burgeoning human potential movement, spreading eastward from encounter and sensitivity groups in California, emphasized a high quality of life, starting with birth. An awake, aware mother and infant were viewed as crucial requirements for entry into a world of expanding human capacities.

A third supporting influence was the fresh awareness of consumers' rights exemplified in the philosophy of Lester Hazell (Chapter Two). As much as the other campaigns, consumerism bolstered the cause of ICEA and ASPO, and led to a short-lived but vigorous health reformation that included medical students in its ranks. Out of frustration with medical and institutional inadequacies, groups like Health-Pac in New York City, the free clinic advocates, and the Medical Committee for Human Rights rose and briefly thrived. An attitude that would have seemed shocking in the compliant fifties gained acceptance — that medical care was simply another commodity and should be scrutinized carefully before being purchased.

However, dust had not settled on these changes when the seventies brought the technical advances that were to wipe out some reforms and render others ineffectual, among them childbirth rights. During the troubled and doubting years of Vietnam and Watergate, the appearance of near-miraculous techniques and instruments was welcomed as a sign that the nation still led the world in medical technology. Fresh and daring techniques appealed to the character of the American consumer who, despite complaints, always wanted "the best, the newest, and the most innovative care available."[24]

Regardless of the new consumerism, Americans still clung to the belief that medical developments sprang out of disinterested scientific research. The truth, according to a government publication on health care costs, lay elsewhere:

> Most of the technological advances in medicine have been introduced to the public in the same manner as any other new product. Providers are reached through paid advertising in their technical journals and through education sessions taught by representatives of the pharmaceutical and medical equipment industry. Consumers learn of innovations through mass media presentations based on information from providers. These methods have promoted the view that purchases of innovative equipment or adoption of new drugs or surgical techniques are justified no matter what they cost or how few people they can really benefit. These advances have been heralded as the reason for improved health status.[25]

In addition, two emerging trends of the seventies advanced the use of the obstetrical technologies: a declining birth rate and a medical malpractice crisis that ironically was a backlash of the consumer movement. Now that American parents were choosing to have no more than one or two children, they expected a perfect child at each birth, and the concept of the premium pregnancy appeared. Claims made by the medical industries led parents to believe that when intervention was used routinely, birth tragedies could not occur. This increased the pressure on physicians who were expected to perform impossible medical miracles. Ironically, however, doctors began to view the technologies not so much as a service to patients, but as protection for themselves and hospital administrators whose best legal defense rested on their use of the newest obstetrical innovations.

In the year 1974 in California, where activities are often considered a preview of national trends, a major malpractice settlement was levied every month. The price of medical insurance increased dramatically, especially for obstetricians whose malpractice premiums rose as much as 400 percent. The medical industries which had developed fetal monitors saw their advantage and, as noted by journalist Suzanne Arms "exaggerate(d) the dangers of labor and the risk of lawsuit to the doctor who fail(ed) to use a monitor." Monitor companies in further pushing their wares employed nurses, she charged, who went around speaking at medical meetings, asserting that all labor was high risk and reminding doctors that a child injured at birth was legally free to sue the attending doctor for nineteen plus two years.[26]

The effects of the malpractice crisis are still being felt in the eighties as obstetricians are threatened with suits over "wrongful birth" (birth of an unwanted child when sterilization or contraception fails) and "wrongful life" (birth of an abnormal child that might have been prevented by diagnosis during pregnancy and genetic counseling). These are concepts which, in the words of science writer Michael Woods, were "unheard of until the last few years."[27] Whether the underlying cause is suit-happy parents, greedy lawyers, or incompetent doctors (More than one lawyer has remarked that the reason there are so many malpractice suits is because there is so much malpractice.), physicians have become notably cautious in their attitude toward birth alternatives, preferring to use tests and technologies on the slightest pretext in case of future legal action.[28]

During this period, two American women actively countered the high-tech trends: Madeleine Shearer on the West Coast and Doris Haire on the East. Both used contemporary research as a basis for their attack; both argued against obstetrical intervention, not simply in a stubborn refusal to accept progress, but in an effort to show how imposing new technologies without adequate research was not always in the best interests of women and their infants. To publicize these concerns, both women held large professional meetings that attracted proponents of normalized childbirth. Shearer used her position as editor and owner of *Birth and the Family Journal* (now titled *Birth: Issues in Perinatal Care and Education*) to persuade medical experts to consider cheaper and safer preventive models of maternity care that would in some cases utilize well-educated midwives. As a physical therapist and ASPO-certified childbirth educator, Shearer was a professional trying to change the health field from within. Haire, however was a citizen activist, an outsider groomed in La Leche League and ICEA as an unpaid volunteer.

## Doris Haire: Lobbyist

Doris Haire began her public life in the mid-sixties as a housewife volunteer in a New Jersey hospital. Propelled by enthusiasm and a love of scientific investigation, she embarked on a path that in the next dozen years moved her from her first project of helping allergic babies by promoting breastfeeding, to a nationally-recognized role as the foremost American lobbyist for pregnant women and their unborn children. In 1972 she produced a monograph on international maternity practices which was so influential that it altered forever the way in which American birth customs were regarded by critics and reformers. Many observers had criticized one procedure or another in labor and birth protocols, but no one had placed all the components of an average hospital birth in chronological order together with their justification and outcome. Few had articulated how such a pattern of intervention distorted the physiology of childbirth so that it was transformed into pathology. And none had had the inspiration to name the pattern by its accumulated effect: *The Cultural Warping of Childbirth.*

The monograph, prepared as a special report to ICEA of which Doris was then co-president with her husband John, appeared with the force of revelation for many of its readers. Some who had felt a growing but unspecific sense of disquiet about certain trends in childbirth saw their suspicions articulated for the first time. One of these was Leena Valvanne, president of the Federation of Finnish Midwives, who came across the monograph soon after its publication.

When I read *The Cultural Warping of Childbirth* I knew something was wrong with the way we were doing things in labor and delivery and started to work for change. Doris Haire set me on course.[29]

Others responded in similar fashion to Doris' work. It became a common reference point with childbirth activists and was translated into other languages and widely distributed among birth educators here and abroad. A decade after its first appearance, *Cultural Warping* remains one of the most accessible and cogent critiques of standard hospital-based birth.

No one who knew Doris Haire as a youngster growing up in northeastern Oklahoma would have supposed she would become the author of any such challenge to American obstetrics nor predicted her subsequent career as a lobbyist in Washington. Her earliest recognized ambition was probably to grow up as quickly as possible, leaving behind the small town of her birth and miserable childhood. The second child of Oda and Sterling Buttry, Doris June was born in August of 1925 in Miami, Oklahoma. Her father, who walked with the rolling gait of the cowboy he'd once been, owned and operated a garage in town. Like his wife, he was born in the state when it was still Indian territory. Both parents were forced to leave school early and go to work.

Spoiled by her father, who clearly favored her over her older brother, undisciplined by her mother, Doris grew up a discontented restless girl wandering the town as she pleased, observing other families, many of whom were better off than her own. She knew it wasn't only money that made families happier, although in her view that seemed to help. There were other elements lacking in the Buttry home—affection openly expressed and rules that meant children were loved. Like other girls of her time, Doris imagined that escape from her home and the dullness of Miami could be found most readily in marriage. The man she dreamed about would have to be intelligent and, if not rich, likely to become so. The possibilities suddenly expanded when World War II brought an influx of young men to military training camps near Miami, Oklahoma.

By then Doris was a pretty and popular girl of seventeen. Few friends or beaus knew that her vision was so impaired that she was nearly blind at short range. Earlier her parents, concerned over her dwindling sight, had taken her to St. Louis for an eye examination. They were told their daughter's congenital cataracts would render her blind by the time she was twenty. The doctors urged the girl to read and learn as much as possible while she could still make out the print; her father agreed, asserting that it was better to be blind than dumb.

In high school, books and blackboards were a hopeless blur for Doris, but she pretended she could see and so embarked on a longtime subterfuge. She made jokes when she tripped over furniture, devised ruses to get others to dial the telephone for her, and masked her growing blindness so successfully she was thought of as simply scatterbrained. In this way she was passed on from grade to grade and eventually graduated with her class. She swam and danced with skill and flirted happily with a number of young men who were courting her. When she enrolled at the University of Oklahoma, she began to use a reader to help her with her studies.

Always in the process of becoming engaged or disengaged, Doris met John Haire while he was stationed at Camp Crowder, Missouri. Their marriage plans were interrupted when John was sent overseas to fight in the Battle of the Bulge, and Doris feared she might never see him again. In an unlikely turn of events, he was posted back to the area the following summer. Soon after this reunion, Doris, clothed in a bathing suit, served him a Sunday dinner after which she told him she wanted to marry right away or not at all. She and John were married that evening by a justice of the peace over the state line in Kansas, thus beginning what Doris has always felt was her true life.

For the New England Haire family, the marriage was something of a shock. Their new daughter-in-law was not only half-blind but by their standards, half-civilized as well. However, John's mother, Pauline Haire, took the Oklahoma girl in hand and taught her what she'd need to know as the wife of a future attorney. John entered Harvard Law School in a special program for undergraduates, and Doris worked at the Harvard Coop, selling underwear. While they were in Boston, another event profoundly changed the course of her life. After an expert eye exam, she was fitted with bifocals, an unprecedented prescription for someone so young. Suddenly, almost miraculously, she could see the world close at hand and could read again. This gift and her growing confidence in the happy marriage led Doris to reconsider her earlier decision never to have children for fear of inflicting on an innocent the unhappy childhood she had thought inevitable.

John's first job was as financial advisor to William H. Vanderbilt whose position of wealth and power was beyond any dream Doris had harbored in Miami. By that time she was seven months pregnant, and old worries had been replaced by new. Supposing the cataracts were hereditary, or something else went wrong? While turning this over in her mind, she came across an article on the Yale natural childbirth program. The journalist reported a concern that drugs given to a pregnant woman might damage the fetus, and Doris seized upon a natural birth as something she could do to ensure a healthy baby. In 1951, choosing to have a baby without drugs or anesthetic was not only novel but difficult. Doris sought advice from Vanderbilt's wife Anne, who had taken a kind interest in her. Later Doris said of her new-found mentor that although she was born rich and married richer, she was also deeply endowed with a sense of service. It was Anne Vanderbilt who taught Doris the rewards and responsibilities of volunteerism and how to give time and money effectively.

Upon hearing Doris' aim for an unmedicated labor, Mrs. Vanderbilt sent her to her own obstetrician, a man kindly disposed toward natural childbirth. The Vanderbilt influence also provided Doris with a private room in the hospital where she could labor in quiet rather than in a ward resounding with the screams and moans of other women. Privilege, however, would not permit John Haire nor any other outsider to stay with her. Relying on a sketchy course in Read breathing and Herbert Thoms' book, Doris had her baby without help or encouragement. During transition, the nurses, their faces stung with disbelief, crowded in the room to watch her. When she faltered and asked for aspirin, they laughed. "Honey, you'll need something more than aspirin to help you now." Refusing anything stronger, she went on doggedly alone and gave birth to a vigorous little girl. This seemed for Doris the first courageous act of her life. If marriage had brought her a new life, the birth contributed a sense of worth. "My ego was born with Betsy."

In 1953 Doris had a son, again laboring without drugs and again on her own. The nurses in the Sarasota, Florida hospital could not believe she was progressing in labor because she made no outcry. When one finally examined her, she was appalled to see a baby about to pop out. In fear that the child would be born without a doctor in attendance, she held Doris' legs together while she shouted for help. Doris knew from her readings that the delay could damage the child and begged piteously to be released, promising that no one would be blamed for the miscalculation. The nurse relented, and the boy was born blue but rapidly recovering. The Haires named him Paul, after Doris' brother.

A second daughter, Anne, was born in 1955 at Columbia Presbyterian in New York City. She seemed healthy, but not long after her birth, turned blue in Doris' arms. She was found to have an irreparable heart defect. In the months that followed, the Haires stood by, numb with grief and fear, while painful procedures were imposed upon the baby in attempts to prolong her life. Doris agonized over the possibility that cortisone she'd taken during an asthma attack early in the pregnancy might have contributed to Anne's defects. She had discussed the drug with her doctor, questioning its safety, but since no ill effects were indicated in the literature, she'd taken it. Now no one could positively assure her that it hadn't affected the baby's heart. At five months, the beautiful little girl died in the hospital. For Doris, grief was mixed with the pain of feeling the tragedy might have been avoided had she known more.

In 1957, the Haires had their last baby in a small, community hospital in White Plains, New York, where they hoped they'd have more control than they'd had with Anne in the huge medical teaching center. The little girl, Lynn, thrived without difficulty. In 1961, the Haires moved to Elizabeth, New Jersey, where John became head of an investment consortium and joined a board of directors serving three local hospitals. Doris embarked on her career as a volunteer when Lynn entered school. She began humbly enough on the pediatric ward where ailing babies encased in bandages were suffering from eczema so severe their hands were tied to keep them from scratching. Instantly curious, Doris poked around among the medical records, looking for something all the babies had in common that might have contributed to the allergies. She discovered none had been breastfed. That fact dislodged a memory of medical advice given to her ten years earlier that she should nurse her babies since breast milk might provide some protection against allergy.

A search of medical literature on the subject produced more evidence of the crucial importance of breast milk, so Doris wrote a pamphlet, "Instructions for Nursing Your Baby," to aid newly-delivered mothers in what now seemed a vital function. She also joined a chapter of La Leche League International where, for the first time as a mother, she discovered women willing to support one another on the matter of child rearing. As a leader, Doris sent a copy of the LLLI manual to Princess Grace and invited her to become an honorary member. The princess accepted, paving the way for her appearance as guest speaker at a convention in 1971, an event which gave the League more welcome recognition. Eventually Doris came up against the League's single-mindedness in the rejection of a sentence in her pamphlet about the occasional use of relief bottles, so she moved on to work with ICEA, taking her pamphlet which became one of that group's most useful and popular publications.

In addition to the lack of professional interest in breastfeeding, Doris found herself questioning other aspects of maternity care. Searching again in medical literature, she could find no scientific justification for the barring of fathers from the labor and delivery rooms, or even for the routinely-imposed shaving and disinfecting of the laboring woman's genitals. This humiliating and uncomfortable procedure, often done when the woman was having hard contractions and needed all her wits and resources to keep going, had been instituted on charity wards early in the century because so many women were afflicted with lice. Soon it became routine for every maternity admission to have the "prep," no matter what the circumstances. However, Doris could find no proof that the absence of family or the prep had actually reduced infection rates as argued or helped the mother and baby in any way.

Operating as a medical detective, Doris continued her investigations of childbirth practices throughout the sixties and became co-president (with John) of the ICEA. In 1971, she visited thirty foreign countries as a firsthand observer of birth customs and gained the data she needed to compile *The Cultural Warping of Childbirth*. When she compared customs with infant mortality rates, she learned that although the United States led the world in technological innovation, it lagged behind twenty-three other developed countries in infant survival. Like her predecessor, Dr. Dorothy Mendenhall, who went to Denmark on a similar journey in 1927, she was told by medical spokespersons from the northern European nations that they didn't interfere with forceps and drugs unless there was a medical need. (See Chapter One.)

Once she furnished ICEA with *Cultural Warping*, its new manifesto for reform, Doris collaborated with John to write a documented manual entitled *Implementing Family Centered Maternity Care with a Central Nursery* (published by ICEA, 1972). By this time the Haires had become experts in the field. As chairman on the Tri-Hospital Board in Elizabeth, John had learned the inner workings of hospital management, and Doris had gathered research for dispelling myths about routines like the prep. Both were aware of the practical barriers against family centered concepts, and they hoped the manual would be used to break through these barriers by offering clear and simple instructions to nurses who might otherwise not know where and how to begin.

In fact, the manual did provide practical direction for many hospitals and health departments even in big-city institutions like Chicago Lying-In Hospital, once DeLee's territory. In 1978, Sheryle Paukert, a maternity nurse practitioner, used the Doris Haire model on Lying-In's postpartum wards which housed large numbers of poor teenage girls from minority backgrounds. These were mothers who allegedly could not possibly be interested in family centered maternity care; and yet Paukert found that they were, if given a chance. It was just such a group, she felt, who would benefit most by having a baby at their bedsides and one nurse (responsible for a total of four mother-baby units) to teach and care for them.[30]

Doris was told by a pediatrician friend that all her knowledge wouldn't impress medical experts unless she could pronounce terms correctly. Taking his advice in 1973, Doris audited a core course in obstetrics at the University of Vermont Medical School. Although she stifled her impulse to question everything, she found herself in a rather chilly atmosphere among the medical students, female as well as male. Doris, who along with other reformers had hoped that women obstetricians would be more inclined to accept ICEA goals, came to the conclusion that medical training itself served as a powerful indoctrination into a system that favored technical intervention.

Medical school raised Doris' consciousness, and she came to feel that the ICEA consumer approach of educating parents to make their desires known was not enough. There had to be a network of friendship and financial backing for professionals devoted to normal childbirth. There had to be money for research on prevention-oriented programs. In pursuit of these goals, the Haires set up the American Foundation for Maternal and Child Health in their home in 1974, later taking the office with them to Beekman Place in New York City where they settled after the children were grown. The foundation was designed to fund projects Doris described as "counterstream" research, outside the popular interventionist trends in childbirth.

After sifting through funding requests submitted to the foundation, the Haires became increasingly convinced that the government, which underwrites the vast majority of medical research in the U.S., habitually gives financial support to high-tech projects at the expense of medicine's most neglected stepchild, the field of preventive health.

In order to test this supposition, Doris wrote inquiries to thirty-five federal agencies. The replies, if they arrived at all, revealed an almost universal cautiousness in tone and often suggested that some other agency must be looking into the matter. Making a summary of these responses and adding strongly-worded interpretations, Doris sent the results to the Senate Subcommittee on Health. Her report moved through various offices helped along by a legislative assistant to Senator Jacob Javits. Eventually, the report resulted in a full senate hearing on obstetric practices in the United States which launched Doris Haire on a professional career as an activist in the nation's capitol.

The first of a total of six congressional hearings that Doris planned and implemented was held on April 18, 1978. She brought medical witnesses, among them Dr. Roberto Caldeyro-Barcia, president of the International Federation of Obstetrician Gynecologists, to testify on the electronic fetal monitor (commonly referred to by the initials EFM) and its role in complicating childbirth.[31] After the hearing, Doris became a frequent visitor in the "lions' dens of Washington" and was often the only woman in a group of male policymakers. She learned to remain pleasantly determined even when professionals, resentful of her criticism, refused to speak to her or recognize her presence in a meeting room. Having many opportunities to observe how matters were conducted in the world of scientific research, government agencies and funding, she confirmed her earlier perception that the system worked to favor certain kinds of research and dismiss or ignore other kinds. Technology expanded because once a project had been funded, both the funding agency and the institution involved in the research had a vested interest in its continuance. As Dr. C. Arden Miller, witness at a state hearing in 1981, pointed out:

> The devil is not technology *per se*, but our current system of medical care which contains strong rewards for expanding the use of new technologies. The fee-for-service reimbursement system and the trend toward specialization favor technology-intensive practice by the physicians; hospitals increasingly acquire new machines and facilities in order to attract and retain physicians and hence their patients.[32]

Scientists working against the mainstream were commonly forced into rear guard action, barking at the heels of advancing technology where excitement and enthusiasm and government funds were generated. Doris saw her mission, in addition to providing what money was available from the foundation, as using all the means at her disposal to bring public attention to the work of counterstream researchers who found it so difficult to get funding support.

In annual meetings titled "Obstetrical Management and Infant Outcome: Implications for Future Mental and Physical Development," she created a forum that brought together experts from child development, medicine, psychology, and physical therapy and exposed them to research on childbirth practices and technology that might otherwise achieve small circulation. This yearly gathering, with the brainstorming and enthusiasm that comes from mixing creative people from various fields, not only disseminated information and provoked discussion, but gave Doris and many others the encouragement they needed to persist in an uphill battle. Gradually the influence of these meetings and the work of the foundation gained in stature. In early 1983, the Pediatric Department of Rutgers' Medical School, the National Institute for Neurological and Communicative Disorders and Stroke, and other groups interested in brain damage problems collaborated with the American Foundation in presenting a conference on "Prenatal and Perinatal Factors Relevant to Learning Disabilities" in Washington D.C..

Prominent among the counterstream scientists Doris brought to public awareness through the foundation were Dr. David Banta on electronic fetal monitoring, Dr. Yvonne Brackbill on obstetrical drugs, Dr. Doreen Liebeskind on obstetrical ultrasound, and Dr. Helen Marieskind on the marked increase in cesarean sections.

## Banta and Thacker Question Effectiveness of EFM

Dr. David Banta, employed by the Office of Technology Assessment, an agency of Congress, collaborated with Dr. Stephen Thacker in 1978 to review over six hundred published surveys on EFM. They found only four studies they considered reliable research. In analyzing these, they concluded that the benefits of EFM when used on low risk mothers were minimal.

The Banta-Thacker report, "Costs and Benefits of Electronic Fetal Monitoring: A Review of the Literature," was published by the Department of Health, Education and Welfare in April 1979, and reprinted in the August 1979 issue of *Obstetrics and Gynecological Survey*.[33] In March of that year it had already been used as the basis of an evaluation made by the National Institute of Child

Health and Development's Task Force on Predictors of Fetal Distress which repeated Banta's recommendations that EFM be reserved for high risk mothers. Subsequently, however, the agency issued a revised document stating that although the committee found no evidence that EFM reduced morbidity and mortality in low risk groups, it recognized that under certain circumstances mothers or physicians might choose to use EFM in low risk situations.[34]

The revised statement was more strongly influenced by the enthusiasm of obstetricians for electronic monitoring than by the Banta-Thacker recommendation upon which it was supposedly based. In suit-happy times, EFM was considered the ideal tool for managing labor and was being used as a standard procedure in many modern hospitals where no matter what her risk status, a woman would be monitored throughout her labor. Often she was told this would save her baby. What she was not told was that the electronic monitor also served the hospital and physician by providing a document which would be useful in possible court actions. The monitor printout on the patient's chart provided proof the doctor had overseen the woman's entire labor, even during the sometimes extensive periods when he or she was out of the labor room.

What was this marvelous new mechanical nurse? External fetal monitoring consisted of circling the abdomen with two belts equipped with devices to record uterine contractions and fetal heart rate. The woman would then have to lie as quietly as possible because motion interfered with the machine's ability to record the incoming signals. In the more sophisticated internal technique, the bag of waters was ruptured in order to insert two catheters into the partially dilated cervix and thread them up into the uterus. One catheter was an electrode, the other a pressure gauge to measure not only the frequency but the intensity of uterine contractions. The electrode was screwed or clipped onto the fetal scalp where it remained for the duration of labor.

Before this technological leap, which many considered the greatest obstetrical advance since the Chamberlens constructed forceps, the mainstay of good labor care had consisted of listening to fetal heart tones intermittently with a stethoscope. In 1917, Drs. Joseph B. DeLee and David Hillis had independently refined the stethoscope by adding a headband, thus leaving hands free for palpating uterine contractions.[35] With the advent of EFM this procedure was eliminated, and heart rate and contractions were measured by the machine.

In 1976, Elliot McClearey, editor of *Today's Health*, an American

Medical Association publication for the lay public, wrote *New Miracles of Childbirth* in which he predicted that EFM would soon be used in all labors. The rationale for such widespread use was the aim of saving certain damaged children who were thought to be casualties of the birth process itself. Those aware of DeLee's prophecy of fifty years earlier that the prophylactic forceps operation would prevent epilepsy, cerebral palsy, and criminal behavior heard a disturbing echo in McCleary's optimistic claim that EFM would save "three out of four babies who otherwise (would) be faced with mental retardation" and would rid society of all the "bad boys and slow learners in school."[36]

Nevertheless, obstetrical researchers forged ahead in studying the significance of fetal heart rate patterns and in identifying variations and decelerations which signaled fetal distress. It was believed that late deceleration indicated anoxia, or oxygen deprivation, a serious danger to the unborn child. If this ominous sign appeared on the monitor screen and persisted for thirty minutes, a cesarean section should be done to remove the baby while it was still alive. This practice, which contributed a good deal to the soaring cesarean rate, was justified on the basis that otherwise, the child would be dead or brain-injured.

There were problems with this reasoning. First, the machines themselves could be inaccurate, especially the external monitor which picked up noises in the room as well as fetal heart tones. Second, EFM produced a very high positive rate, sometimes showing ominous signals when the fetus was not in trouble. The just-sectioned baby in these cases showed no sign of anoxia when it was lifted out of its mother's abdomen. Its Apgar score was high, and analysis of cord blood (pH) was normal. This outcome in which a supposedly distressed infant appeared normal after a cesarean occurred more frequently than people realized. In 1982 it was proven that electronic monitoring showed a 74 percent false positive rate (In seventy-four out of one hundred times that the monitor tracings indicate "distress," there is none.) and a 12.8 percent false negative rate.[37]

However, while admitting that fetal heart rate patterns do not always correlate with fetal condition and infant outcome, modern interventionists made a good case for using EFM by citing the dramatic drop in perinatal mortality from twenty per thousand live births in 1970 to fourteen in 1977, the period during which EFM was introduced and used widely on American maternity wards. In reviewing these statistics, some background is helpful for perspective.

The greatest drop in death rate of infants occurred long before the advent of new obstetrical technologies. In the thirty-five year span between 1915 and mid-century, it fell from a rate of nearly one hundred deaths per thousand births to twenty-nine per thousand. In the next twenty years, the death rate sank to twenty deaths per thousand live births and from 1970 further declined as noted above.[38]

One of the few to disagree with claims that the fall in infant death rate was due to innovations like EFM, David Banta said: "Perinatal mortality is subject to a variety of influences, making it difficult to single out any one factor as causal. . . . For example, during the period that EFM was being instituted in the larger hospitals, perinatal mortality was being influenced by the use of contraception and abortion, better nutrition, better prenatal and obstetric care, patient education and genetic counseling."[39] In 1982, Drs. Howard Brody and James R. Thompson echoed this viewpoint when they wrote in the *Journal of Family Practice*, "Many ob studies are poorly controlled, leading to the conclusion that a particular technology has resulted in an important outcome when, in fact, it might be due to some extraneous factor such as improved nutrition and prenatal care."[40]

Citing causes of infant death is a slippery task. Behind known causes like prematurity lie powerful environmental factors that can produce a high or low infant mortality rate. Kathleen Newland, a statistician, believes medical technology can reduce some infant deaths with crisis intervention but cannot alter the number of deaths caused by conditions like poverty.[41] The WIC Food Program, according to a March of Dimes study, helped to lower the prematurity rate and decrease infant mortality in the seventies, yet EFM proponents take the credit. In a 1980 study of very-low-birth-weight infants "saved" by EFM in a Cleveland hospital, approximately one-third died by the end of the year. Although their deaths were clearly due to birth problems, they were not counted in perinatal mortality figures because they died after the twenty-eight day perinatal period.[42]

A further complication in assessing the value of an intervention such as electronic monitoring is the controversy about what sort of research provides the most authentic evidence. Banta and Thacker's decision to regard most of the EFM studies as unreliable was based on the premise that only a prospective randomized controlled trial represented valid clinical research. While not all agree, it is generally recognized that such trials are the most scientifically accurate method of testing whether an intervention is beneficial or hazardous.[43] By 1982, there were actually five randomized controlled trials on electronic fetal monitoring, all of which supported Banta and Thacker's conclusions that the technology was of little use for low risk women. Their findings had minimal impact on medical practice. In an article titled "The Irresistible Rise of Electronic Fetal Monitoring," Dr. Judith Lumley, an Australian physician and researcher, wrote that implementation of EFM was made on the basis of poorly-done research, but she did not believe that better research utilizing more randomized trials would stop obstetricians from using EFM routinely. Dr. Albert Haverkamp had already produced evidence that women monitored by bedside nurses using stethoscopes had healthier babies than those using EFM (See Note 37.). Despite research, Dr. Lumley thought that doctors would continue to use EFM for three reasons: the strength of the monitor industry, fear of malpractice, and hospital unwillingness to provide a bedside nurse in labor.[44]

## Brackbill: Long-Term Affects of OB Drugs

The second scientist Doris Haire brought as a speaker to a foundation meeting was Dr. Yvonne Brackbill, professor of psychology in the Department of Obstetrics and Gynecology at the University of Florida. When a graduate student proposed a thesis exploring the aftereffects of drugs used during pregnancy and delivery, Brackbill at first discouraged her, assuming that since anesthesia, for instance, had been in use in delivery rooms for over a hundred years, a large body of literature would have accumulated. After discovering to her dismay that there were only scattered studies on such an important subject, she embarked on the largest review of obstetrical drugs in American history. With her colleague, Dr. Sarah H. Broman of the National Institute of Neurologic and Communicative Disorders and Stroke, she took existing data from over thirty-five studies on obstetric drugs, including an NIH Collaborative Perinatal Study which had gathered information on fifty-three thousand children born during the fifties. Selecting out of this group thirty-five hundred healthy children who had been tested at four, eight, and twelve months, and some of whom had been further tested at four and seven years, Brackbill and Broman compared the neurological behavior of children whose mothers had been drugged in labor and those whose mothers had not.[45]

The Brackbill-Broman study, "Lasting Behavioral Effects of Obstetric Medications on Children," showed that obstetrical drugs have harmful effects on behavior over time. Contrary to a general claim that the effects of such medications wear off in a few days or weeks, these researchers said their evidence pointed toward lasting effects that were more noticeable when the child tried difficult learning tasks. This occurred, the researchers explained, because the young brain was still under rapid development and at high risk for damage by drugs taken during birth. Furthermore, the fetal liver and kidneys which are not fully functional during labor cannot efficiently detoxify and excrete drugs. The Brackbill-Broman conclusions were made available to the press in January 1979, following what the *Medical World News* termed a reluctant official release of the one hundred twenty-four page study. "Not since the original surgeon general's report on smoking had such a large-scale study claimed to identify a man-made risk factor threatening to so many Americans."[46]

Once the report was released, there was widespread medical indignation at what some professionals felt was telling tales out of school. A special meeting was convened on March 20, 1979, for Brackbill and Broman to meet with physicians on the Anesthetic and Life Support Drug Advisory Committee of the Food and Drug Administration. After giving their report and interpreting the findings for the group, the researchers were chastised by individual members of the Committee for making the report public, not because it might possibly be justified, or even that it could be in error, but on the grounds that it should not have been given to the newspapers because it would only serve to frighten parents. One doctor said that Brackbill's shrill, strident comments would do more harm than good. In a grim prediction made earlier to a *Washington Star-Ledger* reporter, Brackbill said: "I am very much afraid that they are going to take this study which makes a very clear-cut, cause-and-effect relationship between the obstetric medications and degradations in behavior and intelligence and water it all down."[47]

Long before the report was completed, word of Brackbill's ongoing study had reached Doris, whose concern about drugs in pregnancy and labor had been aroused by the death of her own child in 1955, and she herself began a four-year investigation of the Food and Drug Administration, one of the most powerful health agencies in the government. After becoming a member of the FDA Ad Hoc

Consumer Advisory Committee in 1975, she sounded an alarm about the widespread use of obstetrical drugs. The charge that she issued there and in other government committee hearings was repeated to ICEA audiences: "One in every thirty-five children born in the United States today will eventually be diagnosed as retarded; in 75 percent of these cases there is no familial or genetic predisposing factor. . . . Any drug which artificially changes the mother's blood chemistry . . . can . . . affect the fetus."[48]

It is the parents, not health professionals, Doris told her audiences, who ultimately will bear the burden of decisions made about childbirth; in some cases, the burden may be the lifetime care of a learning disabled or mentally handicapped child. From this position, Doris pressed the FDA to withdraw approval of pitocin for convenience inductions of labor and pushed for the inclusion of warnings about obstetrical drugs on patient package inserts. Learning that, in the case of obstetrical drugs, the FDA considers "a drug risk to be a trade secret," Haire made a final report to Congress entitled, "How the FDA Determines the 'Safety' of Drugs, Just How Safe is Safe?" Among other disturbing revelations about the way in which the FDA made decisions on releasing drugs for public use, Doris wrote that the agency "does not guarantee the safety of any drug, not even those drugs the FDA has officially approved of as safe." Concerning the safety of obstetric drugs, she said the FDA had no automatic process for determining the effect of these drugs on the fetus. Her highly critical report was later distributed by both the American Foundation and the National Women's Health Network.[49]

## Marieskind: Cesarean, the Ultimate O.B. Technology

The third researcher whose work was featured by the American Foundation was Dr. Helen I. Marieskind, editor of *Women and Health* and author of a college text, *Women in the Health System: Patients, Providers, and Programs* (Mosby, 1980). In 1979, Marieskind conducted a Health Education and Welfare Department study on cesareans, titled "An Evaluation of Cesarean Section in the U.S.A.," in which she used the techniques of investigative interview to determine why the cesarean had become, as science writer Michael Woods termed it, "number six on the American surgical hit parade."[50]

Not everyone, Marieskind learned, was disturbed that the cesarean rate had risen from 5.5 percent of all deliveries in 1970 to 20 percent in 1982. "What's so great about delivering from below anyway?" some doctors asked her (reported by Gena Corea in *The Hidden Malpractice*).[51] Indeed, it was not uncommon, she found, for physicians to wonder why women would want the mess and pain of a vaginal birth when they could be put out for surgery. They were also sometimes baffled and irritated when cross-examined by parents who'd been told in labor that a cesarean might be necessary. Why should parents be distressed over the mere loss of a Lamaze birth when it was almost certain that with a section the baby would survive as well as the mother?

The medical profession takes justifiable pride in advances that have transformed the cesarean from a desperation measure of the nineteenth century to a fairly ordinary procedure. Once the most deadly of all operations for the mother, with no anesthesia or blood transfusions to buffer the shock, cesareans were performed only in a last-ditch effort to salvage the infant, although probably not the mother. Until American surgeons found a suture that would hold the uterus together, the "wound was left to nature," meaning organs were simply stuffed back in the abdomen and only the skin sewn up. Infection and bleeding problems frequently caused postoperative complications leading to almost certain death, which remained the case, according to medical historian Harold Speert, until the 1880s when a Dr. Robert P. Harris produced documentation showing that suturing the uterus increased the probability of women surviving the operation.[52]

Although a cesarean is no longer a death sentence, maternal mortality following the surgery is twice as great as that for vaginal births, and there are still complications. Dr. Judith Lumley cited statistics collected by Professor Norman Beischer from 1971–1974 showing that "more than 10 percent of (cesarean) women need a blood transfusion, 23 percent have fever, many have disturbed gut function, and all suffer from severe pain. These symptoms, plus enforced immobilization, limit the caretaking the woman can provide for the newborn infant."[53] In 1977, Dr. Murray Enkin noted cesarean complication to both infant and mother, showing an infection rate of 35–65 percent if the woman had been internally monitored during labor (the catheters having opened a path for infection into the uterus). Preeminent among complications to the infant is the possibility of an ill-timed cesarean producing an infant with immature lungs susceptible to life-threatening respiratory failure.[54] Superimposed upon these serious complications is the post-operative depression experienced by many cesarean mothers. "What is a surgeon's dream come true," wrote feminist Deanne Bunce, "is a mother's nightmare."[55]

Until Nancy Wainer Cohen and Jini Fairley established an organization in 1972 (C/SEC) to support women who had undergone cesarean sections, they were left to deal with pain and disappointment on their own. Few care-givers bothered to reassure their patients that what they were suffering was the expected discomfort of major surgery combined with the ordinary difficulties of becoming a mother. With C/SEC providing the impetus, parents moved to transform the section into a cesarean "birth," and fought for fathers' rights to be present in the operating room to comfort their wives and see their newborns lifted out of the uterus into life. Members also pressed for bikini cuts (low transverse incisions made over the pubic bone) instead of the classical vertical incision from top to bottom of the uterus which took longer to heal and so weakened the organ that it was unlikely the woman would ever be able to deliver vaginally.

Important as these efforts were in fulfilling a need, they did little to answer Marieskind's major question: why had the incidence of cesareans more than tripled during the seventies? The most common response of physicians she interviewed was "fear of malpractice suits if a cesarean was not performed and the outcome was less than a perfect infant."[56] Marieskind's broad-based study uncovered several other reasons, including medical belief that high-tech management would produce a better baby, economic incentives in combination with fear of malpractice, the decline in birth rate that made lucrative cesareans more desirable to doctors, and changing definitions of high risk that made more women candidates for surgical delivery. As an example of the latter, a slight elevation in blood pressure might put the woman into a high risk category; then she might be put to bed or even hospitalized, increasing the likelihood of a series of interventions that often ended in a cesarean.

Marieskind cited serious gaps in medical training as another cause of excess surgery, saying that one of the frequent explanations for the cesarean rate was that "residents were not trained in normal obstetrics and were ill-prepared to manage labor."[57] Student doctors were not taught the nuances of the stethoscope and other simple ways of recognizing trouble in labor, and instead relied increasingly upon EFM and other tests and technologies. Because they almost never sat through an entire labor, they could not recognize normal variations and interpreted every deviation, no matter how small, as a complication. Mothers with breech presentations were routinely sectioned because younger physicians did not know how to per-form a vaginal breech delivery.[58] Although the Marieskind report did not revolutionize medical practice, it caused some activists to reassess their initial enthusiasm for supporting cesarean parents. They suspected that support groups might unwittingly encourage unquestioning acceptance of surgery. Beth Shearer, Director of C/SEC (1983), disagreed: "Criticism is usually offered by women who have had vaginal deliveries. They do not know what it's like to stand up and be sure all your guts are going to fall on the floor in front of you when you're trying to feed your hungry baby."[59]

Shearer was the only childbirth educator on a National Institute of Health Task Force on Cesarean Childbirth, formed in 1981, to determine causes of a rise in cesareans. The resulting report noted "four diagnostic categories that accounted for about 80 percent of all cesareans and 80–90 percent of the rise in the rate: repeat cesareans, dystocia, breech presentation, and fetal distress. The single most important contributor to the rise has been dystocia, accounting for about 30 percent of the increase." Dystocia was defined as a "grab-bag category of general and imprecise terms, including cephalopelvic disproportion (CPD) . . . prolonged labor and 'failure to progress.' " Shearer hoped that the report would alert physicians to the abuses of cesarean surgery and that they would not ignore it in the way they had done with Marieskind's detailed investigation.[60] To lower the cesarean rate, she and C/SEC founder Nancy Wainer Cohen launched an attack on repeat surgeries which account for 27 percent of the overall increase.

Cohen, co-author with Lois J. Estner of *Silent Knife: Cesarean Prevention and Vaginal Birth After Cesarean*, coined the term VBAC, standing for Vaginal Birth After Cesarean. Her book argues strongly that the VBAC is safer than a repeat cesarean which carries two to three times the risk of maternal death and five to ten times the risk of complication. Cohen herself was a model for the campaign, having followed an initial cesarean section with a successful hospital-based vaginal birth and a home birth after that. On the radical side of the cesarean support controversy, she wrote: "Cesarean-childbirth classes are an insult to women. Women and babies need not be subjected to the risks inherent in a major abdominal operation just because it can be a 'good experience.' We see fascination with technology that may someday actually destroy the blueprints for natural birth."[61]

There was, as might be expected, resistance to Cohen's campaign for the familiar reason—fear of malpractice suit if the trial labor ended badly. In demonstrating how the legal situation controlled medical practice, Marieskind earlier cited Cornell University Medical Center which, unlike most other hospitals, had not followed the 1916 dictum of Edwin B. Cragin, Director of Sloan Hospital for Women: "Once a Cesarean always a Cesarean." However, in the wake of the malpractice crises, Cornell Center's policy shifted abruptly, and its cesarean rate leaped from a modest 7 percent in 1965 to nearly a quarter of all births by 1978.[62]

Edith Patton, president of ICEA from 1962 to 1964, observed the VBAC campaign from a unique perspective. She and her husband John, in seeking alternatives to childbirth in the 1950s, came into the sphere of Dr. Virginia Larsen of Seattle (See Chapter Two.). The third of their family-centered births was described by Edith for a 1953 interview in *Ladies' Home Journal* as "the best of the bright sweet moments."[63] But the fourth birth involved a malpresentation, and Edith required a cesarean section, which because of a sympathetic surgeon-colleague of Dr. Larson, was truly a cesarean "birth." Edith was not only awake with John at her side, but she subsequently gave birth vaginally to two more children despite the fact that she had a classical scar in her uterus which, by current standards, would prevent her from even attempting vaginal delivery.

Consumers like the Pattons who pressed for their rights remain relatively rare. Parents are loathe to ask for a second opinion on proposed surgery under the usual conditions, let alone in the midst of labor, especially when told a baby's life is in danger. In the eighties, as more women undergo cesareans or know others whose babies were born surgically, the procedure ceases to seem unusual and slips almost unnoticed into acceptance as an ordinary outcome of pregnancy. In Marieskind's assessment: "The overall effect of the increase is to make cesarean section a routine, expected, 'normal,' procedure."[64]

## Liebeskind: Seeing with Sound, Its Safety in Obstetrics

Dr. Doreen Liebeskind was the fourth researcher to work with Doris. A radiologist and assistant professor at Albert Einstein College of Medicine, Liebeskind and her associates studied the effects of ultrasound on animal cells. In 1979, she developed a new stain to determine ultrasound effects on DNA and growth patterns in exposed animal cells, using ultrasound in doses similar to those used in obstetrics on living women. When she saw that ultrasound-exposed cells changed after twenty minutes of exposure, she carried out further tests, beaming sound waves on the connective tissue of mice and injecting ultrasound-transformed cells into living mice to see if they would develop cancer. Although the transformed cells are considered pre-cancerous, only one out of five injected mice developed cancer in a series of four in-vitro (laboratory based) studies. Still, in presenting her findings to a 1982 March of Dimes symposium at Columbia University, Liebeskind said she felt more research was needed before ultrasound in obstetrics could be declared absolutely safe over a long period of time.[65]

Not surprisingly, this cautious approach was not well received. Physicians and parents alike were awed and delighted by a new technology that could be used in place of hazardous X-rays. Developed originally as sonar and radar to detect enemy submarines in World War II, ultrasound was first used medically to provide heat for orthopedic injuries. In the sixties, diagnostic ultrasound was developed on the principle that sound waves bounce back from a target in the form of echoes that can be measured as they travel through body tissues of varying densities. A probe passing over the body acts as both source of the sound waves and receptor for the returning echoes which are then transmitted to an oscilloscope where they are transformed into a visible pattern on the screen. Since the advantages of ultrasound in obstetrics were apparent, it rapidly found widespread use, thus bypassing the time for randomized controlled trials in which the new technique would have been used for some pregnancies and denied for others.

As applied in obstetrics, the ultrasound probe is moved over the pregnant abdomen to "see" the interior of the uterus (including the fetus and placenta) on a TV screen. With the "sonogram," the obstetrician can detect abnormal growths, identify ectopic pregnancies, locate the placenta, and determine the size of the fetal head. During the process the mother actually sees her baby's image build up as a series of dots on the screen. The procedure is non-invasive, gives immediate answers, and is not uncomfortable except for requiring that the woman have a full bladder to provide a reference point on the screen. Usually she is so pleased and astonished at the miracle of science that produces the image of her unborn child on a screen (and having a complimentary Polaroid snapshot to take home) that she does not question the safety of the technology. Some experts suggest this experience contributes to mother-infant bonding before the baby is actually born and resent suggestions that the procedure can be harmful in any way. To them, Dr. Liebeskind's hesitation seemed unreasonable. What could be bad about such a superb and apparently benign tool?

Ultrasound is a form of energy, but as ultrasound salesmen and technicians point out to both the medical profession and the public, it utilizes only non-ionizing energy, not harmful ionizing radiation as does X-ray. Yet Liebeskind's concern is not unreasonable in light of history, with X-ray a persuasive case in point. Discovered in 1898 by a Bavarian physics professor, Wilhelm Konrad Roentgen, X-ray was such a promising find that, like ultrasound, it was used extensively in medicine for such practical purposes as locating bullets in gunshot wounds and X-raying fractures to set broken bones. It was quickly applied for an ever-increasing variety of conditions by physicians and dentists with good intentions but with little information as to the ultimate effect until the terrible lessons of Hiroshima became known. X-ray, one of the most powerful tools in combating cancer, was discovered to be capable of causing the disease as well.

A number of other unpleasant aspects of X-ray have been uncovered. The younger the subject of X-ray, the greater the possibility of dangerous effects such as carcinogenesis, mutagenesis (changes in the genetic pool), and teratogenesis (harmful changes in the developing fetus leading to absent limbs or alterations in growth and development). Because the risk of harm is greater in a developing embryo and fetus, radiologists currently recommend no more exposure to radiation than 0.5 rad during pregnancy. When maternal doses exceed five to ten rads (when first used in the 1970s, mammograms gave a four-rad dose), some women consider abortion because it is probable the fetus has been damaged. Before this was known, between the years 1920 and 1955, many children were irradiated for tonsillitis, respiratory difficulties, acne, ringworm, and fitting shoes! A review of statistics in 1982 pointed out that a significant number of these children developed thyroid disease in later life. Of the cases of radiation-induced thyroid disease, one-fifth were malignant, demonstrating the carcinogenic effect of radiation many years after exposure.[66]

These facts are used, on one hand, to welcome diagnostic ultrasound into obstetrics as a replacement for X-ray; on the other, to caution against its use before more is known about its effects over several generations. Already some pregnant women are having a succession of ultrasounds for predicting delivery dates. Not only are the woman and fetus exposed unnecessarily to ultrasound energy, but sonograms aren't always accurate for the purpose of fixing gestational age. It is this indiscriminate use of ultrasound in the absence of testing for long-term effects that childbirth educators and women's health activists object to most.

They also worry about its use for another purpose, listening to fetal heart tones with the Doptone in pregnancy and continuously with the external fetal monitor during labor. (Unlike internal monitoring which uses electronic means, 95 percent of external fetal monitoring equipment employs ultrasound.) The argument that ultrasound is safe because it uses harmless non-ionizing radiation is weakened by reports that non-ionizing energy can cause health problems in animals. In 1978, the FDA mandated M. E. Stratmeyer of the Bureau of Radiological Health to study animals exposed to ultrasound in the ranges employed in obstetrics. Stratmeyer found ultrasound exposure caused changes in the development of the animal fetuses and said that ultrasound machine manufacturers should not advertise their equipment as totally safe.[67] In July 1980, the *Carcinogen Information Bulletin* warned that low levels of non-ionizing radiation appeared to lower resistance to disease in animals, thus increasing the probability of developing cancer in the future.[68]

After Liebeskind's 1979 study indicated that more research was advisable to determine safety, William O'Brien, chairman of the Biological Effects Committee of the American Institute for Ultrasound in Medicine, commented in *Ob/Gyn News* that even "if ultrasound is proved to be potentially hazardous in diagnostic doses . . . the diagnostic information coming forth is so phenomenal that to do without ultrasound poses an even greater risk," a statement that sounds like a replay of earlier faith in a specific technology.[69]

On June 12, 1982, *Science News* reported on the March of Dimes Symposium co-sponsored by the Department of Pediatrics and Columbia University's College of Physicians and Surgeons. Reporter Joan Arehart-Treichel forecast a brilliant future for obstetrical ultrasound, saying that in addition to being used for sonograms and external fetal monitoring as it is today, it will be employed in an "ever larger array of fetal health problems." For example, the technique might be used to remove fluid from hydro-cephalic fetuses and to study fetal behavior before birth.[70] In 1983, Associated Press carried a story recommending routine ultrasound for determining the sex of the baby.[71]

Still, some physicians were cautious. In reporting on the same conference in the *Journal of American Medical Association*, Dr. Barbara Bolsen wrote that participants "shied away" from whole-heartedly endorsing the routine usage of ultrasound because of the possibility of "delayed or subtle manifestations, based on the results of animal and in vitro studies in which biological effects have been observed, but which, for the most part, cannot yet be extrapolated to the human condition." She advised her colleagues not to "assume diagnostic ultrasound is innocuous, (but to) keep up with research developments on bioeffects, and use the procedure only when clinically indicated."[72]

Others have warned against the quick acceptance of captivating technologies. Dr. Gary Richwald, medical director of the Los Angeles Childbearing Center, said at a government hearing in 1981, "Technology needs to be very carefully and very appropriately applied if we are not going to have technology substitute for human beings and violence substitute for human care."[73] Such warnings seem particularly significant in obstetrics whose history, perhaps more than that of any other branch of medicine, is a battlefield littered with the tragedies brought about by weapons that seemed miraculously useful at the time. We have only to glance back over the past two decades to see that thalidomide and DES were originally thought to be harmless to the fetus.

In a seemingly more benign instance of mistaken theory, until recently virtually all obstetricians so severely limited pregnancy weight gain in attempts to avoid eclampsia that some women were told they would be dismissed from care if they gained more than fifteen pounds. Rigid diets and diuretic treatments are now believed to produce low birth weight babies and premature births as Dr. Tom Brewer has long claimed.[74] An English medical professor, Phillip Rhodes, provided further perspective during a debate on obstetrical intervention in 1982:

> I would like to remind you of some ghastly mistakes from the past. . . . When forceps and Cesarean sections were first introduced, women and their babies were killed in large numbers when operations were undertaken for inappropriate reasons. Excessive oxygen therapy

for neonates (led to blindness) . . . yet it seemed so right at the time. So did routine X-ray pelvimetry . . . to screen out the possibility of dysproportion. And what about thalidomide? Do we cause damage with other drugs which we give to pregnant mothers in ways we have not suspected?[75]

Professor Rhodes, unfortunately, was one of the few British medical people speaking against the tide of new technology, slower to reach Britain but just as powerful and seductive in transforming obstetrics when it crossed the Atlantic as it had been in America.

## Opposition to High Tech Childbirth in England

Until recently, American activists regarded the British system of maternity care as an enlightened one that included safe home and hospital settings, midwives working in league with physicians, and one type of care for all, rich or poor. This system started to crumble in 1970 when the Peel Committee recommended that all English childbearing women be delivered in hospitals. Once increasing numbers of women were actually in institutional settings, their presence opened the door to accouchement force in the name of research and progress. Five years later, the BBC examined the new management of labor in a documentary that focused primarily on induction, an interference that was used as often as 60 percent of the time in some hospitals. Not only were British medical doctors occupied with an induction craze, but "changing fashion (was) the cause of more extensive use of episiotomy, forceps, vacuum extraction, and Cesarean," according to journalists Catherine Boyd and Lea Sellers.[76]

In another change that represented a major upheaval, England centralized its perinatal services. Women who had formerly received care in small local offices staffed by friendly midwives and family doctors had to travel to urban medical centers. There they were given assemblyline service similar to clinic care for the poor in the U.S.. In the *London Standard*, Valerie Grove, one such clinic patient, told how for weeks she had felt a persistent lump in her upper abdomen which she thought was the baby's head. At every visit which involved waiting for hours in the "lackluster hospital clinic among a mass of disconsolate women," she would see yet another doctor and say she was sure she had a breech presentation. In every case she was ignored, and the doctor would write "ceph," meaning head down, on her chart. After a nurse examined her upon admission to the hospital in labor, she exclaimed, "Mrs. Grove, your baby is upside down." Grove concluded, "All those dreary hours at the clinic had been not only unpleasant but ineffectual."[77] Quoting activist Catherine Boyd, she continued, "Herds of women have to wait like accident victims in casualty when their check-ups could be handled in a more relaxed atmosphere close to their homes."[78]

Resentment reached a peak in 1982 when Professor Ian Craft of Royal Free Hospital ordered an end to flexible policies that favored natural childbirth in that institution. In outraged response, polite British housewives joined with the major childbirth action groups, Association for the Improvement of Maternity Services (AIMS), Association of Radical Midwives (ARM), The National Childbirth Trust and the Patients' Association in a demonstration on April 4, 1982, against the hospital. As small children ran about amongst them, women marched, carrying signs that read, "We Won't Take This Lying Down," "Squatter's Rights," and "Penis Envy Is No Excuse." When the leaders entered Royal Free under friendly police escort, the editors of *New Generation*, the official publication of the National Childbirth Trust, called it an "historic day." *New Generation* added, "It was Sheila Kitzinger who pointed out . . . that women have not taken to the streets before on this issue."[79]

Kitzinger, a well-known anthropologist and childbirth educator from Oxford, saw more in the rally than the journalist's romantic view of "knots of folk moving gently down the road." What she saw was an organized protest of British women who do not frequently join together on a political issue. Encouraging them to further action at the rally, she said that a woman "is not just a container for the fetus . . . she is a person on a journey. . . . When women give birth among friends following the rhythm of their bodies, they usually do better than when their labors are managed continuously by well meaning strangers."[80] Earlier she told a reporter: "the most difficult thing for an obstetrician to do is . . . keep his hands in his pockets instead of interfering every step along the way."[81]

## Sheila Kitzinger: The Splendid Ritual

When journalist Debora Moggach met Sheila to interview her on publication of her latest book *Pregnancy and Childbirth* (Michael Joseph, 1980), she was so taken by the "large fecund looking woman in her loose Indian smock . . . flaxen hair piled high," that she wrote, "one can imagine her working in great generative cycles producing a book every nine months."[82] Indeed, since the five Kitzinger daughters have come of age, Sheila has completed at least one book a year, writing in the early hours of the morning, propped up in a giant four-poster bed as she sips tea. Known for her "psychosexual" method of childbirth, she is a consultant to ICEA and highly admired by American childbirth educators. In England she is spokesperson for natural childbirth, a counselor, teacher and tutor at the National Childbirth Trust, and a research scholar of international reputation.

Before Sheila had given birth to her first child, she commuted between Edinburgh where she was doing postgraduate work and Strasbourg where her husband, economist Uwe Kitzinger, held a diplomatic post. They had decided to have their baby at home — not a radical choice for natives of Britain where, until the 1950s, half of all babies were born in their mothers' beds. For Sheila, the act of bearing a child was perhaps less than she might have anticipated, being quite simple from start to finish and lasting a mere two and a half hours. But in another way, it was much more than she might have imagined: "Overwhelming, preposterous, ecstatic, and quite the most marvelous thing" she had ever done.

When the midwife arrived, she was scandalized to find her patient, a handsome, hearty young woman, squatting on the floor, and immediately persuaded her to climb back in bed which was the proper and fitting place for a laboring mother. Once in bed, Sheila was ordered to push, and although not feeling the impulse, she obeyed. A baby girl tumbled out so swiftly she tore her mother in the process. A doctor was called to sew Sheila up, and dissatisfied with his initial work, he carted her off to the hospital for further repair. When Sheila came out of the anesthesia, she heard him remark to her husband, "There, I've sewn her up quite snugly for you." Later, Sheila would write of the disservice committed by doctors who repaired women's bodies in terms of the sexual services they would provide for men.

In subsequent births, Sheila pushed when she felt like it, lying or squatting as the situation seemed to require. Each labor reinforced the startled perception of sensations which had engulfed her at the first birth. Remembering them afterward and experiencing them again, she came to believe they were essentially sexual in nature. Out of this conviction, combined with reports from hundreds of her students, came a psychosexual theory described in her first book, *The Experience of Childbirth* (Gollancz, 1962), which rapidly became a classic in the field.

After a second pregnancy produced twin girls, Sheila found herself with three children under the age of two. She thought it futile to try to continue in the professional field of anthropology and so embarked on a career as a childbirth educator, or as she phrased it, "threw in my lot with the children." In youth, she had been attracted to three fields: theatre, psychiatry and the Unitarian ministry. Her mother, Clare Webster, was a Unitarian descended from rigorous intellectuals who formed Chapel Debating Societies in the nineteenth century where great and thorny questions were argued in the parlors of ordinary folk. Of women's duty there was no question. It was understood they were the bearers of moral principles and ideals that were to be passed on to the coming generation. Motherhood was a calling that involved far more than mending a child's socks or washing a face; it was a duty of utmost significance.

Sheila's father, a tailor-weaver whose Scottish family had wandered into southwest England, was also a doer of good in the world and shared his wife's humanist values, except for pacifism. The horrors of the Great War turned Mrs. Webster into a pacifist, a position from which she never deviated despite many arguments with her Methodist husband. During World War II, Clare astonished and outraged her neighbors by inviting German prisoners into her home in an attempt to unite enemies. Among her friends in the small town, she numbered a psychiatrist, a Unitarian minister, and other intellectuals given to discussing Jung, Freud, Maria Montessori, and A. S. Neil. She also had a following made up of women trapped in unhappy marriages or ill-timed pregnancies, or barren women who came to her for solace and advice. Young Sheila, noticing the whispered and tearful consultations, developed a respect for the depth and inner workings of women's lives. Human beings, her mother said, should do something about what they were given in life; it was morally wrong to simply sit back and accept whatever happened. She wanted Sheila to have the education she had missed, having been forced to make a living at thirteen, and she taught the girl at an early age always to strive, for without striving there was no purpose in life.

Sheila attended Bishop Fox's School for Girls in Taunton, Somerset, becoming head girl, and then she studied drama for a year in

Bristol, qualifying for a teacher's license from the London Guildhall School of Drama. She read widely, moving from one enthusiasm to another—Kierkegaard, Simone Weil, Shaw, Ibsen, Martin Buber, Olive Shreiner and the World War I poets. Her aptitudes lay in journalism and psychology, but she studied social anthropology at Ruskin and St. Hugh's Colleges in Oxford.

Sheila met Uwe Kitzinger while she was still at Oxford, and they were married in the interval between her first degree and postgraduate work. When Uwe accepted the post in Strasbourg, France, and Sheila went north to Edinburgh to teach and continue research, the Kitzingers began what was to be a long-term pattern of pursuing a marriage in two countries. The first daughter, Celia, was born in Strasbourg, and Sheila started teaching childbirth education classes in their living quarters there. Later Uwe returned to England to the Oxford School of Management Studies, and the couple lived in an Oxfordshire cottage where the twins, Tess and Nell, were born followed by two more daughters, Jenny and Polly, all born at home. When the cottage overflowed with little girls, the Kitzingers moved into a sixteenth-century manor house that had been part of Henry VIII's settlement on his fourth wife, Anne of Cleves. There, in a vast sitting room with a stone fireplace carved in Tudor roses and ceiling beams salvaged from ancient sailing ships, Sheila taught classes and played with her children, telling them stories and fashioning dramas in which they all performed.

Since Uwe was often abroad, she managed to raise her daughters on her own much of the time. The local welfare office sent a series of teenagers to act as mother's helpers, but they were sometimes more in need of mothering than the Kitzinger children, and Sheila often found herself doing social work at home to keep the mother's helper in good shape, rather than being relieved of household duties. Nevertheless, she was able to build a career in childbirth education and develop theories that grew into the first book—written, out of necessity, in the early morning hours before the children arose.

In proposing a strong sexual component to birth, Sheila was in agreement with Niles Newton who also cited the event as an expression of feminine sexuality, although the two women had not exchanged ideas. From the beginning, Sheila took issue with the French reformers, Lamaze and Vellay, for advocating distraction as the means of coping with labor pains. She thought the basic tenets of the psychoprophylactic method were mistaken. She did not object to preparing for the reality of pain, knowing from her mother who had sometimes attended women at childbirth that labor pain could be the most severe a woman would ever endure. However, she did object to the use of distraction in reconditioning theories that taught women to shift their attention away from what was happening to them and to focus it instead on breathing patterns. In redirecting consciousness, Sheila proposed, not only was the perception of pain removed, but also the body awareness necessary for full participation in the childbirth experience—"the intense and thrilling sensations of the descent of the baby's head," and the accompanying feeling of the vagina gradually opening, "like the uncurling petals of a rose."[83]

*Experience* offered different methods of relaxation based upon Sheila's training in the Stanislavski Method of acting, involving a series of mental images combined with touch instead of speech. Touch relaxation, Sheila's best known contribution to the lexicon of childbirth preparation, requires the partner to assist the laboring woman by using hands to signal the release of tension in place of command or admonition. With this method, the partner guides the woman into a relaxed state in which she flows with the innate rhythm of labor instead of detaching. Far from resisting contractions, she "greets" them by loosening herself and concentrating upon a mental image. If she tightens and feels pain, she is reminded by her partner's gentle hand upon her body to release herself again.

This process enables a couple, assuming the labor partner is also the sexual partner, to heighten mutual awareness and enhance their relationship. Sheila was criticized later, notably by American poet and feminist Adrienne Rich in the essay "Theft of Childbirth," for assuming that every birthing woman had a husband to coach her, certainly a common assumption at the time.[84] Rich may have been unaware that Kitzinger had always been keenly alert to discrimination against unwed mothers and by the seventies, was including women from changing family structures such as lesbian mothers and their partners in her childbirth classes. Publication of this first book (and others to follow) brought Sheila many letters from women grateful to have someone finally acknowledge the emotional and psychological aspects of giving birth.

In 1965, recognizing his wife's growing career and need to do research, Uwe Kitzinger accepted a temporary academic chair in Kingston, Jamaica. There Sheila, in collaboration with the Medical

Research Council at the University of the West Indies, wrote a study of sex, pregnancy and childbirth among Jamaican women, where fragments of West African traditions from a former slave population mingled with those of eighteenth-century European plantation owners. In West Indian villages she saw the grafting of both influences onto native beliefs about childbirth. There was the midwife or "nana," a highly respected personage, whose relationship with the pregnant woman began long before the baby was born and continued long afterwards in a net of female comradeship. The midwife knew firsthand the circumstances of the mother, what she ate, how she cared for herself, and what her worries were; she made this knowledge part of her service during pregnancy and birth.

Later, as a recipient of the Joost de Blank award (1971–73), Sheila studied Jamaican women after they had emigrated to London where they abandoned the old ways of the nana. Through an honorary fellowship at St. Mary's Hospital, she attended clinics for Caribbean women and accompanied visiting nurses and pediatricians on house calls where she found immigrant women eager to discard their traditional culture. In their need to identify themselves with new and modern ways, they were grateful for any attention from the white-coated experts, no matter how patronizing.

Through a reputation as lecturer and teacher on childbirth, Kitzinger was invited to other countries where she again observed how women in transition from old ways into new experienced their childbearing. In South African villages, she saw ancient methods of coaxing the laboring woman to open her body that were in sharp contrast to management in modern hospitals a few miles away, where women of differing language groups were crowded together in wards and cared for impersonally by staff more interested in their physical signs than in belief systems that might influence the course of labor. In the sixties, Sheila visited East German maternity hospitals where Pavlovian theories had somehow been interpreted to mean strenuous conditioning treatments, including a post-delivery treatment for pelvic floor relaxation in which streams of cold water were sprayed between the legs of uncomplaining, stoic women.

Sheila Kitzinger began to see that the manner in which a society treated its childbearing women provided a powerful indicator of what the culture valued, and it was important, first of all, to ascertain who controlled the place of birth. In the United States where hospitalization was universal for childbirth, male doctors were clearly in charge and traditional wisdom discarded as nonsensical folklore. This, Sheila felt, impoverished the lives of women and cut the ties between generations. Furthermore, eliminating a continuity of female support made women more vulnerable to professional control and more likely to accept what was given them without question.

Sheila's detachment as an anthropologist enabled her to point out the unspoken messages that establish superiority or inferiority of participants in such a matter as childbirth. Clearly, the laboring woman in a modern hospital is made aware of her subservient position during the first few moments at the admitting desk. As a person who has given up her autonomy by becoming a patient, she is expected to obey those in charge of her well-being. This is part of what Sheila called the "splendid ritual," Western society's version of the birth ceremony. It was to her credit as an actress that she could dramatize both old and new rituals, as she did for an appreciative audience in Palo Alto, California, in 1979, in one of many appearances sponsored by the ICEA.

A heroic figure with the healthy face of an English girl, lined but still rosy, and dressed in a golden kimono, blond hair piled on top of her head, Sheila acted a scene from a Caribbean revivalist church where women worshipped through song and dance. She rocked and gyrated in rhythm, stunning her audience with a dance that put the West Indian women in touch with the mysteries of their common past and opened them to a shared future.

With equal drama, she described a different sort of ceremony, the rites of high-tech birth. The patient, dressed in hospital-issue gown, lies in bed with catheter in one arm and others inserted through her vagina into her uterus and infant so the contractions and fetal heart rate can be recorded on a machine. Communication between woman and man is limited since she is immobilized and he is intrigued by blips on the monitor. Already the woman has undergone initiation into the patient role by ritual shaving and cleansing. She undergoes further humiliation in a delivery room filled with surgical equipment and people by masked figures.

> When an obstetrician isolates with drapes the lower half of a woman's body, it becomes *his* sterile field. But it is clearly neither his nor, because of the juxtaposition of vagina and anus, sterile. It is a convenient fiction however by which he asserts his rights and insists that the woman keeps hands off her own body, which becomes out of bounds.[85]

None of these procedures is designed to prepare either mother or father for the responsibilities of parenthood, nor is there an expectation that during birth they ought to receive such support. After the baby is delivered, while the woman lies supine with her legs in stirrups, the newborn is presented to her so that bonding can take place. While Sheila has no quarrel with the significance of research done by Klaus and Kennell, she finds it ludicrous that the infant is applied to the mother for a specified interval following a high-tech birth, on the assumption that natural forces will magically take over, as if bonding were some sort of "sticky plaster."

For the next few days in the hospital, the woman is treated as if she were a mindless child needing constant supervision and correction in feeding and caring for her baby. Then, still fresh from these "rites of humiliation," the new parents are dismissed and sent home to manage as best they can on their own. Sometimes they will have been covertly evaluated by those professionals that Sheila scornfully refers to as "baby bopper detectives." These are psychiatrists and social workers in the hospital who attempt to identify potential child abusers by certain subliminal tests. The tragedy of child battering, she asserts, can be better alleviated by offering more attention to women during pregnancy, especially those existing on meager means, isolated in urban centers and bereft of family and community ties. These circumstances, added to the splendid ritual, might well prevent some women from forming strong maternal connections with their children—but they are seldom considered by the experts.

However, the splendid ritual affects all women no matter what their economic status, Sheila believes. Through its procedures, women are removed not only from their personal identities but from the actual birth and are drawn into medical rites as zealously guarded as any ceremony in the old cultures. Step by step, the woman is divested of all that is familiar in a bionic environment where she is totally dependent on strangers who themselves rely on machines for information. Inherent to this new ritual is the belief that the machines are faultless, truthful, and indispensable in the delivery of a healthy baby.

For all her appreciative description of native birth rituals, from the nana in Jamaica weaving her network of support to the African witch doctor blessing the ground at birth time, Kitzinger does not advocate return to a romanticized past. Well aware that birth in pre-industrial societies was often terrifying and dangerous, she asks that Western cultures revive only those rituals that will grant the new family an identity and respect presently withheld, and that the birthing woman retain sufficient power and control over her body to move into her new maternal role with some degree of confidence.

These themes underlie all the Kitzinger books: *Experience of Childbirth* (Gollancz, London, 1962), *Education and Counselling for Childbirth* (Ballier Tyndall, London, 1977), *Giving Birth: Parents' Emotions in Childbirth* (Sphere, London, 1972), *Women as Mothers* (Fontana, London, 1979), *Birth at Home* (Oxford Univ. Press, 1980), *Diary of Pregnancy* (Grossett & Dunlap, 1981), *The Complete Book of Pregnancy and Childbirth* (Knopf, 1980), and *Woman's Experiences of Sex* (G. P. Putnam Sons, 1983). Sheila has functioned as such a productive writer partly because of her ability to organize a working party, drawing on the knowledge and skills of professionals from various backgrounds.

Out of one such gathering came *The Place of Birth* (Oxford University Press, 1977) which Sheila co-edited with John A. Davis. The impressive compilation of reports and essays contains epidemiologist Iain Chalmer's work on the absence of proved causal relationships between improvements in perinatal statistics and modern techniques such as induction, forceps, and cesarean sections. Variation in their use from country to country, according to Chalmers, indicated little agreement as to their advantages. He added that early criticism of interventive obstetrics had come not from concerned doctors like himself but from people like Sheila Kitzinger who had reported adverse effects of induction in 1971, and whose monograph *Some Women's Experience of Induced Labor* (National Childbirth Trust, 1975) had helped bring pressure on Britain's Department of Health and Social Security, which subsequently launched its own study leading to a diminished use of induction in Britain.[86] In America, Doris Haire's work on the consumer committees of the FDA also resulted in lower induction rates.

To prepare *The Good Birth Guide* (Fontana, London, 1979), Sheila put an ad in a London paper, asking for stories of hospital births and received hundreds of letters in response. She sorted out the comments, compared them with official statements of policy issued by each hospital mentioned by a letter writer, and then gathered them all into a consumer's guide to services for labor and delivery. The impact of the guide was so powerful that some administrators wrote her, insisting that they'd improved their services since the report and requesting she update the book so that they wouldn't lose patients.

## The Politics of Episiotomy

In 1981, again after requesting responses from numbers of women, Sheila published another monograph through the Trust: *Some Women's Experience of Episiotomy*, and edited eight papers on the subject which were published as *Episiotomy: Physical and Emotional Aspects*. All these works underscore the unpleasant effects of the surgery while noting its almost universal popularity among American and British obstetricians. Sheila had earlier noted that in the United States almost 98 percent of childbearing women received routine episiotomies, and those who missed them did so only because they delivered before their doctors got the scissors well in hand.

Kitzinger has recorded that nearly all women complain bitterly about the pain of episiotomy and its association with difficult marital relations following birth. Yet doctors defend the surgery because it shortens the second stage of labor. This is alleged to prevent damage to the fetal brain from "pounding the perineum" (see DeLee's recommendation in 1920) and to prevent over-stretching and trauma to the mother's vagina and pelvic floor. Medical texts insist that without episiotomy, women will be stretched to the point of developing vaginal relaxation with subsequent prolapse of the uterus and bladder that causes leaking urine and other problems in later life.[87]

In 1972, Doris Haire reported that no research existed to prove these theories and that, in fact, they were medical myths. There simply were no data showing that routine episiotomy reduced the occurrence of pelvic relaxation, and "shortening the second stage of labor by performing an episiotomy when there was no sign of fetal distress has not been shown to be beneficial to the infant. The scientific evaluation of seventeen thousand children . . . indicates that a second-stage labor lasting as long as two and one half hours does not increase the incidence of neurological impairment of the full-term infant who showed no signs of fetal distress."[88]

But there was another reason for doing routine episiotomy, and that was that the procedure would serve men in keeping the vagina snug for intercourse. In an essay titled "Natural Childbirth and the Reluctant Physician," Shelly Romalis identified the viewpoint of male doctors toward the operation. "The less stated reason, although one taught in medical schools, (is) that the tightening of the enlarged vaginal opening will prove more sexually satisfying to the man . . . the final stitch is thus often referred to as 'the husband's stitch.' "[89]

Whatever the rationale, episiotomy is so popular among obstetricians that it is the most common of all surgical procedures performed on women. Typically, the operation is done without asking the delivering woman whether she wants it or not, or even suggesting that it might be elective. Yet episiotomy involves more than a minor cut made at the bottom of the vagina and, as Kitzinger found, makes intercourse more painful for the woman for a time. The incision, made with scissors, extends deep into layers of muscle that include a layer of erectile tissue and blood vessels associated with sexual responsiveness. Male doctors seldom express sympathy for post-episiotomy pain since they consider the surgery's benefits to outweigh the risks of any alleged discomfort, but at least one woman doctor has challenged her colleagues on the subject. When asked by fellow obstetrical residents why women don't like episiotomies, Michelle Harrison, author of *Woman in Residence,* responded:

> "Because it feels like a violation."
> "That's ridiculous . . . It's important to do them. Don't women understand they will stretch too much if they don't have one?"
> "Well, Neil, first of all, it has never been proven they will stretch more. Second, it's painful after delivery, and third . . . I'm saying that many women feel they're being mutilated without having any choice in the matter."[90]

However logical or persuasive her argument, Harrison knew she was wasting her breath. Physicians, influenced by medical texts that state unequivocally the absolute necessity of episiotomy, find it almost impossible to revise that view. They persist with the practice in spite of strong evidence that most well-nourished women who have been trained in relaxing the perineum so that they can release muscles during labor, and who deliver without having their legs forced apart in stirrups, and who follow their spontaneous bearing-down urges will ease their babies out gently without sustaining serious tears.

Drs. David Banta and Stephen Thacker reviewed medical literature on episiotomy in the same way they checked on EFM research.[91] In 1982, their government-sponsored study supported claims made by

Doris Haire, Sheila Kitzinger, Niles Newton, and Dr. Rosemary Cogan ("The Unkindest Cut") that episiotomy operations do not prevent jagged tearing of the mother's tissues, nor spare the infant's oncoming head, nor minimize or prevent brain damage. Furthermore, the surgery does not enhance sexual pleasure or prevent vaginal relaxation in later years.[92]

In addressing the politics of episiotomy, Sheila, like Doris Haire, keeps chipping away at the unnecessary rites of medicalized birth. Neither woman bows to male medical authority, and neither woman blanches in the face of organized opposition, no matter how well-funded or established. Because of the relative security of their positions, they do not have to maneuver as do reformists within the health system who know their jobs and careers are at stake. This freedom makes each of the women a formidable opponent in whatever battle she chooses.

Doris Haire has continued to march into the lions' dens of Washington where, on one occasion, she cheerfully outraged a group of lawmakers by saying it was "better to have an ironing board in the labor room than a fetal monitor. At least then a woman could be on her feet and (would) have a brighter and more alert child for it." In 1976, she joined the feminist movement through the National Women's Health Network, having come a long way from her girlhood dreams of making life work by finding the right man. Still in league with ICEA and other childbirth groups, she joined forces with the more demanding organization, offering her skills at lobbying and her knowledge of health law and regulation to further its aims as set forth in *Resource Guide on Maternal Health and Childbirth:*

> We, as women, by choice and necessity are becoming more active participants in the protection and promotion of our own health. Increasingly we are finding that the health services we need are unavailable, inadequate, and sometimes dangerous. . . . [93]

Sheila hopes, through her writing and teaching and a new (1983) BBC series on childbirth preparation, to counteract the current monopoly of knowledge by professionals. In a society that appears awestruck by the cabalistic rituals of institutionalized medicine, Sheila works for the time when each woman is confident enough to look her doctor in the eye, to use his given name when he uses hers, and to ask forthrightly for the information she needs in order to make sensible judgments about her own condition. In this effort she appears to be carrying out her mother's belief that each of us is responsible for our choices in life and that "we must strive to challenge all that is unjust, unloving and unwise in the order of things."

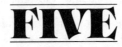

# FIVE

# The Midwife Question

Women have always attended other women at birth . . . and they always will. When women want and need services that institutions can not or will not provide, other women will create them.[1]

Norma Swenson

The appearance of the lay midwife or domestic practitioner in American homes has raised all the old arguments over the midwife question. Who is to educate and regulate her, and how? What place does she hold in American health concerns? And what right, if any, does she have to function at all? These questions are being debated in courtrooms across the country as midwife after midwife is arrested for practicing medicine without a license.

## Old and New-Age Midwives

The ancient and long-respected profession of midwifery has often been under attack in the past.[2] Midwives practiced at the risk of their lives from the late fifteenth century until well into the seventeenth, when thousands of women were accused of witchcraft and burned at the stake in what might be termed a "campaign of terror directed against the female peasant population."[3] According to historians Barbara Ehrenreich and Dierdre English, the ruling classes and churches used fear and terror as the means of keeping peasants in line. Priests resurrected and refined discarded beliefs about partnerships with the Devil unleashing enormous hidden powers capable of bringing harm to the innocent. Detailed procedures for identifying and prosecuting witches were laid out in a book written by two German Franciscan monks. *Malleus Maleficarum*— The Hammer of Witches—published in 1484, achieved rapid distribution due to the just-invented printing press, and for nearly three hundred years remained the official blueprint for a fiery persecution whose primary target was women.

The midwife, according to the *Malleus*, was the "worst offender" of all women accused. As she went among her neighbors, dispensing herbs that could reduce a fever or stop a hemorrhage, she represented a dangerously independent and inquiring spirit, one likely to incite resistance to authority. Midwives also had ready access to material long believed magical—umbilical cords, amniotic sacs, and placentas. With these substances, a midwife might easily enter into a pact with the Devil. She might transfer womens' pain to men, render men impotent, sell the soul of an infant, perform abortions or help dispose of those newborns whose care and presence was unendurable. In short, she could protect women from the righteous punishment of church and state. Even when she did not use her knowledge for evil, she was still suspect by virtue of offering health care to those the church and ruling classes felt were best left to God's ministrations.

When the witch craze finally ebbed in the late 1600s and midwives were free to practice without fear of being put to fiery death, some taint clung to them still, marking women who secured their own knowledge about the human body through observation and practice and who used that knowledge to provide healing for others. Even in the twentieth century, a whiff of witchery lingers about anyone seriously pursuing a study of herbs and home remedies, and midwives are often still accused of having malevolent intentions. They have seldom been referred to in literature or medical texts in any but an unfavorable light, often by reference to the infamous Sairy Gamp, an inept and drunken midwife in Charles Dicken's *Martin Chuzzlewit*, "whose nose in particular was somewhat red and swollen.... She went to a lying-in or a laying-out with equal zest and relish."[4]

English medical historian Anthony Smith, ignoring the long established precedent of trained midwives in Great Britain, refers instead to an earlier historian's description of midwives as "ragged old harridans who traveled from house to house like tinkers with their old-fashioned labour chair and filthy hooks hanging from their belts."[5] Thus, he joins other contemporary writers who, evaluating the role of midwives in obstetrical history, have invoked the image of Gamp as though she were a real person with hundreds of descendents plying a "poorly regulated craft varying greatly in experience, skill, cleanliness, integrity, and sobriety."[6] There is seldom, if ever, an acknowledgment that the same description could have been applied equally well to all other practitioners of the healing arts of the time.

Midwifery has in some areas of the world remained a respected occupation. In many European countries it has been integrated into the health establishment. In Holland and Scandanavia, for example, midwives offer a consistent and comprehensive maternity care that makes them highly regarded, well-paid members of the community.

In the early years of the American colonies, midwives were accorded a similar regard, for they provided an essential service available from no other source. A Mrs. Bridget Lee Fuller, passenger on the Mayflower, acted as the Pilgrims' "Physiction and Chirurgeon." In 1630, Trijn (or Tryntje) Jonas had her passage to the New World paid by the Dutch West India Company. In return, she was to attend the settlers' wives in childbirth and thus ensure the colony's growth.[7] There are other occasional references to midwives during those early years, often honoring them for the vital function they served; however, there was still some concern, particularly in Puritan New England, that midwives not overstep the boundaries proper to their sex and status.

Seen as a threat was a woman named Anne Hutchinson, a scholarly person and member of the female intelligentsia in Boston. She was cousin to the English poet John Dryden and wife of a successful merchant who supported her through her troubles with the authorities. Known as a "woman very helpful in the times of childbirth, and other occasions of bodily infirmities, and well-furnished with means for those purposes," she believed that God's grace could be found in every person, rather than being reserved for the favored few, a leading religious doctrine of the day.[8] In addition to her meddling in theology and causing dissension among the clergy of the Massachusetts Bay Colony, she was also criticized for holding organized meetings of women in her home. Feeling against her mounted even further when it became known that she had been present at the birth of a deformed child. Accused of witchcraft, she was called before a religious synod and banished from Boston. She and her family fled to Rhode Island where she was later killed in an Indian raid. Popular opinion ran so strongly against her that church bells in Boston rang for twenty-four hours in celebration of her death.

The fates of her women friends were likewise grim. Dr. Jane Hawkins, who had attended the birth of Mary Dyer's deformed child, was warned by the authorities not to "meddle in . . . physick, plaisters, or oyles" because of "notorious familiarity with the Devil," while Mary, unwisely returning to Boston some twenty years later, was condemned and hanged for her Quaker beliefs.[9]

For the most part, however, midwives continued their work unremarked in the colonies until well into the eighteenth century when the increasing number of physicians in settled areas stiffened competition. Doctors casting about for ways to expand their practices noted the advantages of attending women in birth. It was observed that once a woman had been safely delivered by her doctor, she was likely to call on him for all medical services for the family thereafter.

By 1730 or so, many doctors had gained a further edge over midwives, at least in the eyes of middle and upper-class women— the possession of the new highly-touted birth extractors or forceps. The question of why the new instruments remained almost exclusively in the hands of male doctors and surgeons has been discussed repeatedly but never completely settled. It is certain that midwives, whatever their inclinations, were barred from training in anatomy and surgery. They had no professional organizations to assert their rights to share in new developments, and few of them could afford the forceps, even if they learned to use them. However, there was also a deeper philosophical barrier between women and men birth attendants, most eloquently articulated by Elizabeth Nihill in her *Treatise on the Art of Midwifery: Setting Forth Various Abuses Therein, Especially as to the Practice with Instruments.* Her chief target was the well-known William Smellie, an English doctor, self-taught in the new skills of obstetrics, who is credited with breaking the monopoly of female attendants at birth. He promoted male obstetrics among barber surgeons and anyone else who could pay the fees for his practical courses in childbirth and use of forceps. Smellie and his followers, Nihill charged, used the instruments only for "dispatch," to hurry the birth process at whatever cost in pain and possible injury to the woman. Jean Donnison, author of a definitive history of English midwifery, chronicles Nihill's complaint that the male practitioner "was so adept at concealing his errors with 'a cloud of hard words and scientific jargon' that the injured patient herself was convinced that she could not thank him enough for the mischief he had done."[10]

Although Nihill's work did serve to bring the issue to public attention in England (there was no similar midwifery outcry in America) and to promote discussion of the wisdom of interfering in birth, it was clear that the ability to hasten what was for many women a long, agonizing process, often made the men and their instruments seem preferable to women who used only their hands. In the middle of the nineteenth century, doctors gained a powerful advantage over midwives in their access to anesthesia. During this period, women seemed to suffer inordinately in labor, perhaps due to weariness from constant childbearing and general poor health exacerbated by tightly-laced corsets. The popularity of drugs grew rapidly, and barely a decade after Dr. Simpson experimented with chloroform in Scotland, an American physician, Tom Metcalf, noted that the query that almost always greeted his arrival at the bedside of a laboring woman was, "Have you brought the chloroform?"[11]

Access to drugs and instruments gave inarguable advantages to doctors over domestic practitioners, but otherwise, medical handling of childbirth remained crude. The brand of medicine practiced then, before the scientific discoveries of the late nineteenth century, was of the sort usually called heroic, often employing violent means to cure diseases: terrible purges, scalding baths, emetics, and bleeding. A laboring woman might have leeches applied to her perineum, or her veins might be opened to ease her pains, allowing her to bleed until she fainted which served, after a fashion, to blot out the pain. Infusions of alcohol or vinegar might be forced into the uterus in an attempt to halt postnatal bleeding. Doctors used the same drastic methods in treating most conditions, leading a contemporary observer, William Cobbett, to describe the treatments of heroic medicine as "one of those great discoveries which are made from time to time for the depopulation of the earth."[12]

In the first decades of the nineteenth century, there was an American revolt not only against this intolerable form of healing, but against authority at all levels. With Andrew Jackson, a champion of the common man, in the White House, a nationwide drive for class equality led activists to crusade for women's and working men's rights and for a return to traditional means of healing. Health leaders rose to prominence, preaching the need to take responsibility for one's own health through diet, exercise, and balanced living. Ladies' physiological societies offered classes on female anatomy and self-care. There were warnings against bad food and air and restrictive clothing and the chronic invalidism then beginning to afflict women of the upper classes.

To the consternation of the so-called regular doctors, thousands of Americans transferred their health care to homeopathic practitioners who were concerned with the whole body. Popular theorists included Sylvester Graham who ate whole grains and abstained from liquor and drugs entirely, and Samuel Thomson, an herbalist and lay healer who had been instructed in his youth by a midwife. Thomson, the most important of the Popular Health leaders, supported womens' rights and advocated that only women, whom he considered natural healers, should attend other women, most certainly in childbirth.

Fueled by the national enthusiasm for democracy, the Thomsonians and other reformers were astonishingly successful. In a brief period, 1830–1840, they managed to overturn most of the medical licensing laws in the country, opening the doors to healers of all persuasions and training. However, due to various factors including internal quarreling and dilution of the movement by quacks and patent medicine peddlers, Popular Health began to lose strength by mid-century. In 1847, the regular doctors having seen their profession slip into a craft in which anyone could practice and profit, organized themselves to insure their survival. The American Medical Association was founded primarily to increase economic benefits to its members, some of whom were in reduced circumstances as a result of mass defection of patients to other healers. For the rest of the century, doctors in the AMA worked to reestablish licensing laws designed to secure their exclusive right to the practice of medicine. Membership in the AMA came to be vital to a career, and members were strongly urged to run for office on the state and local level in order to influence legislation.[13]

Among the homeopaths and other irregulars, midwives were a special target for elimination. Conventional doctors feared that if upper-class women once again turned to midwives for delivery, they might also seek them out for other ailments.[14] During this period of increasing prudery, the doctors had the additional problem of persuading modest women that attendance by a male midwife was appropriate and seemly. Their overwhelming success in doing so was due to various changes in the social atmosphere, one of which was the declining need for womens' domestic labor in the wake of industrialization. Working-class women left home often to work in factories and mills, while middle and upper-class women were left without any vital function except that of bearing children. Under enforced leisure and tightly-laced, unhealthy fashions of the latter half of the century, women of privilege slipped into chronic invalidism, requiring frequent medical visits. Doctors advised their patients to avoid mental and physical strain of any kind lest they fall victim to various ailments centered in the female organs. "Society had assigned affluent women to a life of confinement and inactivity, and medicine had justified this assignment by describing women as innately sick."[15]

A stream of books warned women against seeking education for fear of upsetting their delicate physical balance. Dr. E. A. Clarke's *Sex in Education* (1875) maintained that intense mental effort by women damaged their reproductive capacities and that higher education for women thus endangered the human species. In another volume, *Perils of American Women*, Dr. George L. Austin held that infection of the female ovaries was responsible for "marked effects upon the brain and nervous system. indigestion, spinal irritation, many forms of neuralgia, headaches, mental irritability and insanity."[16]

Writer-lecturer Catherine Beecher who advocated that a woman's place was in the home was, nevertheless, concerned about the poor physical state of many housewives she interviewed in a variety of locations in the nation in 1855. Taking a poll in her immediate family, she found that of nine married sisters or sisters-in-law, all except two were "delicate" or actually invalids. Of fourteen married female cousins, all were ailing or disabled.[17] No doubt some invalid women were using sickness as a form of birth control or were suffering from forceps injuries. Whatever the cause, the conditions contributed greatly to a growing dependence on doctors for all sorts of needs.

By the end of the century, middle and upper-class women were convinced of the superiority of physicians for childbirth, while the midwife continued to practice her craft, out of sight, among poor and working-class people. In the eighties and nineties, great waves of immigration from Europe brought old-world midwives to American cities in significant numbers. In New York City, two of five births in 1900 were attended by midwives, a number large enough to attract attention, especially during a period of welfare reform instigated largely by middle-class women. When some of these groups in New York publicized the high infant mortality rate, doctors responded by blaming midwives. (See origins of Maternity Center Association in Chapter One.)

In 1910, Carnegie money funded a national survey on the state of medicine, which resulted in the Flexner report, celebrated since as the means by which medicine was finally upgraded into a reliable, regulated scientific profession. Among other recommendations, the Flexner report advised that a campaign be mounted to "drive midwives out of the maternity field and promote obstetric physicians, raising obstetrical fees so the field would attract able men."[18] There was another motive less publicized but equally important in the campaign to eliminate midwives. Obstetricians, like members of all other specialities, were often inadequately trained. The fault lay not only in schools with wildly varying standards, but in the lack of clinical experience. If poor women continued to seek midwives for their confinements, student doctors would have no one on whom to practice. One doctor stated the problem openly in the Journal of the AMA: "It is at present impossible to secure cases sufficient for proper training in obstetrics since 75 percent of the material otherwise available for clinical purposes is utilized in providing a livelihood for midwives."[19]

The attack on midwifery became part of a growing move toward hospitalization for all childbirth, a move supported not only by the doctors who originated it, but soon by women themselves. In a period of veneration for all things scientific, hospitals were extolled in the popular press as the modern preferred place in which to give birth. Only women who couldn't afford doctor's fees, or worse, women too ignorant to know better, called in a midwife. In the next decades, the word "midwife" was hardly ever used without the prefix "ignorant and dirty"; and racial and ethnic slurs were hurled without fear of refutation. Midwives were called "mammies," "grannywomen," "hags," and "crones." One critic pointed out that since many were immigrants, they weren't even real Americans and certainly not appropriate members of the health profession.[20]

So well did this campaign work that the number of midwife-attended births in New York City declined from two-fifths in 1900 to one-tenth by 1932. In the same period in the nation, midwife deliveries dropped from 50 percent of all births to 12 percent in 1936, and 80 percent of these took place in the South.[21] However, maternal mortality rates did not plummet during that time as expected by those who had so readily blamed midwives. In 1930, the New York Academy of Medicine conducted a survey of all maternal deaths in the city. The results which were, to the indignation of the medical profession, printed in 300 newspapers in the U.S. and Canada, showed that 60 percent of the deaths of mothers were preventable, and that a majority of those (61.1 percent) had been caused by physician error.[22]

Some four decades later, after the midwives had been virtually eliminated, medical historian Dr. Neil Devitt made an exhaustive survey of documents on the New York midwife to see whether she deserved her unsavory reputation.[23] He concluded that while contemporary surveys showed the preparation of midwives to be poor, it was not much worse than that of physicians of the time, and some immigrant midwives had received excellent training in their own countries. Novelist Gay Courter found support for his conclusions in research for her novel, *The Midwife*.[24] There was evidence that many midwives, whether immigrant or not, were willing to avail themselves of whatever educational services were offered. Devitt uncovered the reports of Dr. Josephine Baker who had attempted to upgrade and educate midwives in New York City in the face of medical hostility. Her work showed that the midwives of 1900 who had delivered 40 percent of the babies were responsible for only 22 percent of maternal deaths from sepsis or infection, whereas physicians in charge of the other 60 percent of births were responsible for 69 percent of the maternal deaths from infections. Dr. Julius Levey of the New Jersey Department of Public Health did a study in Newark in 1916 which showed that midwives not only had better birth outcomes than physicians, but they were sometimes charged unfairly with a death, "even where it appeared that the result was due to unnecessary interference or negligence on the part of the doctor."[25]

Nevertheless, the attack on midwives with the AMA in the lead continued unabated. When citizen reformers proposed legislation providing for maternal child welfare, including funds for childbirth education (Sheppard-Towner Bill, 1921), the AMA responded with a fusillade long-remembered for its bombast. An editor of the *Illinois Medical Journal* claimed this bill was the work of "endocrine perverts, derailed menopausics and a lot of other men and women working overtime to destroy the country."[26] Considered the first act of enfranchised American women, the legislation passed, but funds meant for improving midwifery and holding prenatal classes were eventually diverted to medical research when doctors convinced legislators that childbirth was a disease and, therefore, properly their province.

A few midwives continued to work, mostly out of sight in rural areas where they presented no economic threat to physicians. Some of these women, often called grannies, have left written or oral records of their work. In *Hillbilly Women*, the author tells the story of one: "Aunt Molly Jackson was a midwife in Eastern Kentucky during the twenties. She delivered babies and doctored families of union miners. One day, after seeing countless small children die of pellagra, Aunt Molly robbed a company store at gun point, taking enough food to feed a few families."[27] David Stewart introduced another traditional midwife at a NAPSAC conference: Minnie Mae Farr from Marvel, Arkansas, the mother of fifteen children born at home and a practicing midwife in her community for twenty years. As a young girl, she had gone with her mother to births and been struck by the feeling that she had a calling for midwifery. From that time on, she sustained a devotion and commitment to the art, and in old age had an excellent record of service. On January 1, 1980, Minnie Mae, along with all other lay midwives in Arkansas, received notice from the state that her profession was no longer legal.[28]

For most Americans, the midwife had been discredited long before. A nurse midwife, attempting to establish practice at Roosevelt Hospital in New York City in 1964, noted the still potent effects of the smear campaign. "It (midwifery) conjured up images of old women with dirty hands and stained clothes, delivering babies in hovels while burning herbs at the foot of the bed."[29]

The counterattack was long in coming, and when it finally appeared, heralded by the new-age midwives, it was accompanied by some profound changes in American life-styles. Among these was a movement back to the land, where dissidents attempted to live on their own, growing food, building houses by hand, and caring for one another's ailments as people had done in the past. The reappearance of neighbor attending neighbor in birth was a natural part of these new attempts to live in old ways. As the movement gathered force, fed by other evolutions in thought and attitude of the late sixties, established institutions attempted to reassert their control. In California, where counter culture parents were choosing home births, the new-age midwifery flourished but always on the edge of the law and always under the threat of civil action.

The first lawbreaker to come to national attention was Raven Lang, a Santa Cruz midwife and artist. To the defenders of scientific medicine she was an outlaw, while to those who heralded a return to the ideals of Popular Health she was a heroine of legendary proportions. It was Raven Lang who called together the other midwives of Santa Cruz County, women practicing in fear and isolation among the mountain communities. Out of this gathering in 1972, the famous Birth Center came into being.

## Raven Lang: Lay Midwife

Raven was born Patricia Lang in 1942, the daughter of Emma Parenti Lang who'd run away with a cable car gripman and gone to live with him in the Irish section of San Francisco. In a few years, the marriage collapsed, and Emma assumed total responsibility for raising the children in the Mission District where Pat and her brother attended St. Peter's Parochial School and were spared worse than they got on the streets only by grace of their Irish name.

Although she never knew him, she had an anarchist grandfather, Elpidio Parenti, who emigrated from Pisa, Italy, to America with the intention of organizing workers. He was jailed in New York City with Alexander Berkman and later named his eldest daughter, Raven's mother, for Berkman's lover, the celebrated feminist free-thinker and midwife, Emma Goldman. After Parenti was released from jail, he took his oldworld wife and their five daughters to California, organizing in the coal mines of Utah and Wyoming as he traveled West. In San Francisco, the family settled in North Beach.

Pat was a dreamer, a studious and devout little girl who believed she could fly into heaven if she wanted and converse with the angels. All of her childhood she suffered bouts of asthma and other illnesses. At nine she lay paralyzed briefly with spinal polio, and when she was twelve, fell into a long and inexplicable decline that was diagnosed as malingering. Her mother was told her daughter would recover once her periods started. Finally, Pat collapsed on the street with rheumatic fever. After hospitalization, she was put to bed at the home of her Aunt Lina, the youngest and most successful of the Parenti sisters. In her brusque way, Lina encouraged Pat to use her sharp mind, to become a bookkeeper like herself, perhaps something better.

In high school, Pat joined a troupe of avant-garde dancers, and developed such skill at shorthand that she won a competition and was offered a highly paid job as part of the prize. She turned it down, saying she did not want to become someone's secretary; she wanted to go to college and major in science. Her mother, scraping for survival in the neighborhood laundry, had little patience with her arty and unrealistic daughter whose aspirations, she felt, did not match her station. After a year or so at City College, Pat's unconventional life and friends made living at home impossible, and she moved out on her own. When her money ran out, she had to take just the kind of job she'd so blithely turned down earlier.

Her skills won her a desk in the front offices of the Bank of America, but she didn't last long there. A penchant for dancer's slippers, long full skirts and unshaved underarms, coupled with reluctance to run back and forth serving coffee to the male executives marked her for transfer to an interior office where training films and manuals were produced. Her feminist supervisor, Anita, recognized the young woman's ability and soon taught Pat all she knew about technical writing and layout. When Anita left her job, Pat was not promoted, as the two women had expected. Instead, she was directed to train an unqualified young man as her new supervisor. Pat rebelled and covertly removed all the training material from the files.

Earlier she had established a friendship with a French janitor at the bank, a man in his sixties who shared the young woman's enthusiasm for the literature and language of his homeland, and they often ate lunch together. When Pat was called before the bank's personnel board, she fully expected to be castigated for hiding the files and refusing to train Anita's replacement. Instead, the issue was what sort of books she read and the nature of her friendship with the janitor, who was considered a union agitator. Members of the board demanded the right to examine the contents of Pat's purse, actually a wicker basket containing her ballet shoes, lunch, and texts for night-school classes. The board suspected it might also contain union propaganda for secret organizing among bank employees. Outraged, Pat grabbed up her basket and, advising the board members "to go fuck themselves," she whirled out of the Bank of America forever, her mane of long black hair flying behind her.

After the fiasco at the bank, Pat returned to college, this time as an art major. At twenty she was no longer the homely dark Italian child among the Mission Irish but an increasingly attractive and able young woman with respect for herself and her talents. The following summer she took a temporary job with an ad agency where her supervisor in art production was Ken Kinzie, a divorced man who had custody of his half-grown children. Soon he and Pat were deeply involved with one another, planning to share an artistic life and a commitment to human service. When they married in 1966, California was on the verge of a cultural revolution, and the Kinzies were markedly influenced by many changes going on around them. Ken went to teach at an alternative school in the Santa Cruz mountains while Pat took over as best she could the care of her step-children and continued studies at the San Francisco Art Institute where she had a scholarship. Then, a leader at an encounter group at Ken's school singled Pat out, charging her with being too mannish and having neglected her essential femininity in copying tough women. She should, he insisted, learn how to become a woman by having a baby.

In an abrupt turnabout typical of the progress of her life, Pat quit her part-time newspaper job, became pregnant, and dropped out of school at the end of the semester when the Kinzies moved to Ben Lomond, a mountain community in Santa Cruz County. For the first time in her life, she lived in the country. In a meadow of uncut grass surrounded by redwood forests, her senses expanded with pregnancy, and she felt herself merging with nature. The "mountains of Ben Lomond," she would write in *Birth Book*, "gave me a trust in the natural order of things and helped me to experience the integrity of the universe."[30]

When Pat Lang—she'd kept her own name after marriage—walked out of Stanford University Hospital with a son in 1968, she had questions about childbirth she would spend the next decade trying to answer. In what had been the most powerful experience of her life, her body, tuned by the discipline of the dance, responded with a will and knowledge of its own. She wondered whether all women had the same sort of body wisdom buried under layers of fear and expectation of pain, and whether instincts might be inhibited by the clinical atmosphere of a hospital birth, causing women to hold back instead of allowing their bodies to work.

The same sort of innate knowledge marked one of her early encounters with her infant son, Lang. She knew from hospital routine that he would be last when the babies were brought from the nursery for feeding. As the first baby, which couldn't be hers, was brought onto the ward, crying with hunger, she felt her breasts tingle and her uterus clamp down. A new shift of nurses had changed the order, and the crying baby was her own child, as her body had already so clearly informed her. The incident made a deep impression and caused Pat to wonder what initiated and sustained motherly feelings. Later she would observe other mothers responding to their newly-born infants and learn that a gentle birth at home promoted intense interest in the child, not only on the part of the mother and father, but in all those present at the birth. She would also see a few women for whom the act of birth, no matter where it took place, did not inspire the characteristic rush of affection that pediatrician Marshall Klaus would call "bonding."[31] When Klaus and his colleague John Kennell began to conduct studies on maternal-infant bonding in the seventies, he sought out Pat for her special knowledge of the way women responded to their infants when they could handle them immediately after birth.

Pat's childbirth experience also caused her to question the infallibility of medical doctors and their practices. She was given an episiotomy as was usual, but the aftereffects seemed unusually severe. She suffered a good deal of pain when she sat or even walked after Lang was born, but no one bothered to explain why this might be so. Taking things into her own hands while she was still in the hospital, she managed to get a look at her chart and discovered the obstetrician had cut clear through to the rectal sphincter, a mistake that's not uncommon and is rarely admitted to the patient.

Putting her anger into action once she was well, Pat trained herself through reading and discussion with a young doctor, who had been doing home births until forced to cease by his colleagues, and became the first childbirth educator in Santa Cruz. She held classes and accompanied women to the hospital, coaching them through labor and encouraging them to remain fully conscious. Soon she was an ubiquitous figure on the labor wards of Santa Cruz, dressed in boots and jeans, her long hair tied back, as she stood by a hospital bed assisting her students with breathing until they were wheeled away to the delivery room and the doors closed behind in Pat's face. While she awaited the outcome, she recorded in a large hardbound book every response of the woman to her labor.

Until a particular birth in 1970, Pat Lang felt that women should always have their babies in hospitals. She hoped that with her instruction, they would have a better time of it, would ask more questions, and would have more control over what happened. With this in mind, she convinced those parents who wanted a home birth to go to the hospital. It was this sort of woman that Pat accompanied one morning at a point when she was sure the labor was progressing well. The young woman, excited and confident about the birth although she would have preferred staying home, was told by an admitting doctor that she'd have her baby by lunchtime. However, the woman's obstetrician was delayed and gave orders by telephone that she was to have an injection of narcotics to slow the labor. At noon she was given another shot, and Pat sat troubled by her sleeping student until mid-afternoon when the obstetrician appeared. Pat was ordered out of the room for a time. When she returned she found an IV needle inserted in her student's arm—containing a solution of glucose for energy, the doctor said. The sluggish labor picked up amazingly, and soon the woman's uterus was woody-hard with steady contractions although she could feel little, due to an injection in the vaginal area. Insistently questioning the nurses, Pat learned that pitocin, the artificial hormone used to start and stimulate labor, was dripping into her student's veins. Nurses came and went, constantly checking vital signs. One of them, listening to fetal heart tones with a stethoscope, detected abnormal rates. The doctor was hastily fetched, and the young mother, weeping over her ruined labor, was hustled onto a gurney and rushed to the delivery room where her baby was hastily extracted with forceps.

To Pat, the pit drip was both a shock and a revelation. Now she knew that certain procedures like a hasty episiotomy or a labor stopped and started with drugs could be done for someone else's reasons and not solely to improve health in the baby or mother.[32] In the seventies, the pit drip was merely part of an everyday routine to keep the hospital running like a factory, and some doctors timed their patients with pitocin so that they attended mainly daytime deliveries instead of being wakened in the night.

The granddaughter of an anarchist found her just cause. Exposure to the pit drip transformed Pat Lang into Raven, although her new name came later. One day when she was walking near the cabin where she lived in Ben Lomond, the name of a child she'd delivered seemed to fly onto the path before her. It was "Raven," namesake of a bird of prophecy, known in the old days as a messenger of the gods. The name had seemed right for the little girl at first, but when her skin turned rosy pale and her dark hair was replaced by blond wisps, her parents gave her a rosier name. Pat went in to ask them for the gift of the old name which they granted. So Pat Lang became Raven, and the name suited her as if she never had another.

One of eight midwives in the area, she had by then become a true empiric, studying books but learning most directly from experience. She learned to detect an unborn baby's heartbeat by ear and to feel the child in the womb with highly-skilled hands. As she gained in experience, others came to learn from her, and she began to make a name for herself as a midwife. When more and more women in the long dresses of the counterculture went to the midwives instead of to Santa Cruz doctors, physicians in Santa Cruz became alarmed at what they proclaimed was a public health menace. The local medical society held a meeting which Raven and a doctor friend attended, hoping to contribute to the discussion and thus gain some measure of physician collaboration. However, they were not allowed to speak, but had to sit and listen while they were condemned and the doctors arrived at a plan for controlling midwives. It was decided in a unanimous vote that the obstetricians would refuse prenatal care to anyone intending to have a home birth. They would no longer see such women at all for blood tests or any sort of care during pregnancy and would not follow them up after the home birth. These threats the doctors hoped would bring recalcitrant parents back to their senses and into medical offices and hospitals.

But the threats only fed insurgency, and in a meeting with the other midwives, Raven, who was by that time recognized as their leader, took the women a step further, urging them all to provide the needed prenatal care themselves. Following a scheme for self-help inspired by Jerry Rubin's *Do It Now*, they would learn how to set up charts, take blood pressures, and test urine. They would learn how to estimate a due date and then under the tutelage of Kitti Lokas and other interested nurses, they would give the pregnant women who came to them the protection of prenatal care.

Out of this gathering, the Birth Center came into being in 1971. The midwives attended regular study sessions and took turns offering their own homes for unique all-day clinics. Pregnant women, their partners and midwives sat on the floor, sharing with one another their concerns and confusions, and easing a common dread of childbirth. The midwives offered their knowledge freely to one another and to their clients. Some time during the day, each one would take a woman into a bedroom for a careful physical examination. Over a period of weeks each pregnant woman would have had a session with each midwife and then could choose the one she wanted to attend her. In the process of submitting to judgment made by the people they served, the midwives gained in both humility and personal confidence.

As the known leader of the lay midwives, Raven had been under surveillance not only by admirers but by local and state authorities alerted by Santa Cruz doctors. Aware of this, Raven decided now was the time to show the community what they had accomplished, especially the excellent birth outcomes demonstrated in data gathered by a Stanford medical student, Louis Mehl. Mehl had fully expected to find the homebirth results inferior to those in the hospital, but instead the data showed both a lower rate of death and a much lower rate of complications.[33] The Birth Center midwives decided to sponsor a day-long symposium to be held on the land where the Kinzies lived. Invitations were sent to the medical community, to parents, and to sympathizers. On March 25, 1972, over a hundred people crowded into a dome built for the occasion. There were professionals in jacket and tie, and coordinated pantsuits mingling with women in long velvet and lace trimmed skirts and sandaled men in tunics.

In the dome, people testified that home birth could restore human experience lost in a technical world. A child coming into life in its own home was welcomed by family rather than strangers. Giving birth back into women's hands provided an intense experience for the participants. For some, there was transcendental joy at the moment of birth that purified and strengthened the bonds among them. The power and awe of childbirth was manifested in large black-and-white photographs at the entrance of the dome. A half-naked woman leaned down to take a bloody child from between her legs. Midwives knelt on the floor to support a child's head straining for release from the mother's body. A crouching woman gave birth, her anus bulging, the infant's head just emerging from her vagina. Near the photos were statistics compiled by Mehl to show how well mothers and infants had done under the care of the midwives. The numbers combined with the beauty and stark reality of the photos blasted the belief that the Santa Cruz midwives were ignorant and untrained women.

Then parents explained why they had chosen midwives, trying to avoid what Raven would describe in *Birth Book* as "outrageous insults of mind and body and intellect when the baby is taken from the sounds and smells . . . that are its birthright."[34] The atmosphere turned political when Raven challenged Palo Alto obstetrician Don Creevy to give the midwives more training because no doctor in

Santa Cruz would help them for fear of losing hospital privileges. Raven had always sought medical help when it was needed, but in the climate of suspicion that had developed in Santa Cruz, local physicians refused help to her and the other midwives. For this reason she had cautioned her clients to assume the responsibility for any risk in a coming birth. Parents at the Symposium agreed they had decided to take that risk and knew, however small the chance, that someday there might be a tragedy. Still, they believed they were safer from infections and mistakes that occurred in hospitals. The day ended on a note of affirmation and celebration for out-of-hospital birth. With a few objections from indignant hospital personnel, the audience honored the midwives who had guided so many parents into taking responsibility for themselves and their birthing experiences.

In all its triumph, the symposium was the beginning of the end of the Birth Center. Too much had been made of the midwives' success, and too many parents began seeking them out. For Raven also, the times were in a distressing transition. Long-time supporters moved away; men she knew were in jail for refusing to serve in Vietnam. In Santa Cruz, a university town known for its activism, both revolutionaries and rightwingers were carrying guns. Dismayed by this atmosphere, Raven accepted an invitation in the summer of 1972 to help establish a medical program providing care for Indians and others isolated in the interior of western Canada. A few days after she arrived, the socialist party came to power, and Raven fell in love with the country and its government, astounded that she was getting what seemed a generous wage for doing what she wanted. When the short-term job was over, she came back to California temporarily and put all her energies into completing *Birth Book*.

Early the following year, traveling in a car filled with boxes of the newly-published book, Raven and Ken and Lang moved to Canada where they were to live for the next three years. In Vancouver, Raven founded another birth center before moving on to Vancouver Island to teach and work as a midwife. During this period, the Kinzies, whose needs were always modest, were mainly supported by sales of Raven's book. One of the first volumes on childbirth, demonstrating the profound changes wrought in upheavals of the sixties, *Birth Book* — a "collection of intimacies . . . proselytizing for home birth . . . " was eagerly taken up by members of the counterculture everywhere.[35] A large format paperback beautifully designed by Raven and Ken, it was illustrated with the stunning photographs from the symposium. Included were the story of the Birth Center, a short history of obstetrics, and an essay on imprinting and maternal affection, but the heart of the book was a collection of narratives of homebirths movingly recounted by the participants themselves. To the establishment, *Birth Book* seemed an unwarranted attack on modern obstetricians, professionals unused to being put on the defensive in the face of criticism by lay persons. There is a story that the celebrated Leboyer, proponent of gentle birth, happened to pick up a copy while on a visit to the U.S.. After leafing through Raven's book for a few moments, he dropped it with a shudder, pronouncing it the work of the devil.[36]

## Midwife Arrests in California 1974–1982

The Birth Center midwives and their growing clientele in the Santa Cruz area had been viewed with increasing disquiet by the authorities on both local and state levels. Something had to be done to curb them, and the California Department of Consumer Affairs, acting on behalf of the Bureau of Medical Quality Assurance, was the agency chosen to do the job. The department bided its time until one of its own investigators became pregnant, and then in Raven's words, "they used her body to entrap the midwives."

The investigator and a man acting as her husband disguised themselves in hippie clothing and went to the Birth Center for prenatal care early in 1974. On March 6, the investigator called the Center saying she was in premature labor. Although Jeanine Walker and Linda Bennett had been uncomfortable about this client and her history all along, they went to the address given them to ascertain her condition and, if necessary, to accompany her to the hospital. Two men also dressed as hippies greeted them at the door and pressed money into their hands. Immediately afterward, the men revealed themselves as undercover agents and arrested Walker and Bennett for practicing medicine without a license.

Meanwhile, police were ransacking the home of midwife Kate Bowland, which was the current site of the Birth Center. Bowland telephoned Raven who happened to be in California for a visit, and Raven notified the press before coming over to observe the bust. She stood in Kate Bowland's front yard, watching as police carried out bandages, blood pressure cuffs, stethoscopes, and even diapers as "evidence." A detective showed her a photograph of herself and asked if she could tell him where to find the ringleader. Raven, unrecognizable in a fur hat, shook her head and went off to alert sympathizers and organize a midwife defense group before she returned to her work in Canada.

The three arrested midwives were charged under Section 2141 of the State Businesses and Professions Code. Their attorney, San Francisco feminist Anne Flower Cumings, immediately filed a demurrer, claiming that the charges against her clients were too vague to allow her to prepare a defense and that the state law against practicing medicine without a license was too broad and failed to define what is illegal. Her stand was that if pregnancy were defined as a normal process rather than a disease, then attending women during labor could not be called practicing medicine. This was to remain the major defense tactic over many months, as the case moved from one court to another.

After a municipal judge denied her petition, Cumings moved to superior court where Judge Harry Bauer accepted her argument and ordered the district attorney to file an amended complaint charging the women with specific acts that fell within the restrictions of the state code. "I gather," he wrote, "that these women are being charged with being midwives, but the complaint doesn't tell me that they are charged with midwifery."[37]

Back in Santa Cruz Municipal Court, the district attorney accordingly made an amended charge accusing the three women of "undertaking to assist and treat a woman in childbirth . . . and treat for a physical condition."[38] Although midwifery was still not specified as illegal, it was this last phrase which was eventually to seal the case for the prosecution, but that was several years in the future. Cumings repeated her petition for demurrer—a plea for dismissal on the grounds that even if the accusations are true, they don't constitute a crime—and again carried it to superior court. This time she lost. Her argument was based partially on repeal by the state legislature in 1979 of a law providing for licensing of midwives. If there were no means by which they could be licensed, she said, the midwives were free to practice on their own. Somewhat predictably, Bauer did not agree with that interpretation and argued that even if pregnancy were not a disease, the state had a right to insist on close medical supervision.

Cumings sought relief in the appellate court and won a round when Judge P. J. Molinari ruled in favor of the midwives, accepting the definition of pregnancy and birth as not pathological. District

Attorney Bill Kelsay vowed to take the case to the supreme court, and if he lost there, he remarked bitterly, " . . . feel free, ladies and gentlemen, to go out and deliver anybody's baby and suture them up."[39]

The supreme court handed down a twenty-page decision, concluding that while pregnancy was not an afflication or ailment, it did fall under the jurisdiction of Section 2141, requiring a license for the treatment of "injury, or mental or physical condition." Nearly three years after their arrest, Bowland, Walker, and Bennett were again liable for prosecution for practicing medicine without a license. But the district attorney who had initially charged them announced in December of 1976 he would drop the case, saying it had achieved its purpose in the supreme court ruling, and besides, the Birth Center had since closed. Actually, the Center did not finally disband until 1978. Its closing was partially due to a change in the women who soughts its services. When malpractice premiums soared in the mid-seventies, doctors increased the fees for prenatal and delivery care from three hundred fifty dollars to over seven hundred dollars. Women on welfare could no longer afford hospital birth and so turned to the Center, but not all of them had adequate background for taking on the responsibility and discipline necessary for a home birth without drugs. In addition, the midwives, with the assertions and counter-assertions of the arrests still ringing in their ears, had even less hope of finding physicians to back them up in emergency. Raven's original organization had operated on the principle of consensus among equals. Now in an atmosphere of stress, the lack of leadership worked against the Center's survival. Eventually, the midwives disbanded and either ceased practice or worked quietly underground on their own.[40]

In spite of the fact that the midwives had actually lost, Anne Cumings felt the case had aided their cause, and there was some evidence to support her view. The legal proceedings which were well-covered in the press, had exposed the injustice of allowing a medical monopoly to control childbirth and had aroused favorable publicity from all over the country. (In one of the hearings, supporters of the midwives entirely filled the courtroom, and the overflow spilled out on a lawn all the way down to the banks of the nearby San Lorenzo River.) But if the case had aroused supporters, it had also alerted those who wanted to see midwifery outlawed in California. These people knew that someday, somewhere, a woman would hemorrhage or a baby die in a midwife-attended birth at home. They knew also that midwives were exposed to public view and lacked the institutional curtain of silence that shielded mistakes in hospital birth. They hoped that when the inevitable occurred and the woman was charged and convicted, the midwife question could be settled at last.

What they waited for took place in San Luis Obispo, California, in July, 1978, when Marianne Doshi could not resuscitate a newly-born child. She immediately summoned an ambulance and the attendants, after reviving the child, transported her to Mt. Zion Hospital in San Francisco where she died shortly afterward. On July 6, Doshi was arrested with another midwife, Cherilee Virgil, a registered nurse who had attempted to deliver a woman at home and, misjudging the labor as arrested, had brought the woman to the county hospital emergency room. Some local authorities apparently suspected that the two women were members of a criminal midwifery ring responsible for an unknown number of backyard burials, although no evidence of such infant deaths was ever found. Virgil was released on a misdemeanor charge, but Doshi was jailed, accused of second degree murder and of practicing medicine without a license. The parents of the dead infant, Robert and Christine Gannage, refused to press charges and stood by Doshi, insisting she had done all she could to help them and their baby. Nevertheless, the district attorney sustained the accusation, and the case moved toward trial.

Doshi secured the services of Anne Cumings, veteran of Santa Cruz. This time, rather than defending on the basis of a definition of pregnancy, Cumings sought a classification of the cause of the infant's death. She asked whether death had come "at the hands of another" or from natural causes. It had already been determined that the baby, Amy Gannage, had died from a knotted umbilical cord. The midwife had not tied the knot, Cumings asserted, nor had she intended harm in any way; therefore, death had occurred from natural causes.

The district attorney, Gregory C. Jacobson, rebutted this argument on the grounds that the infant's death was a classic example of what could happen during a home birth in the absence of a fetal monitor. The monitor would have shown a dip in the fetal heart rate pattern, and if that had persisted, doctors would have performed a cesarean and saved the baby's life. The defense countered that the monitor was not always accurate, nor were its tracings always accurately interpreted. Babies still died of cord problems in hospital deliveries, and no one could say whether or not the Gannage baby would have survived.

This argument convinced Judge Richard Kilpatrick who declared Marianne Doshi innocent of the charges. The evidence, he said, showed him that the baby had indeed died from natural causes. In a subsequent interview with the press, Kilpatrick rebuked San Luis Obispo doctors for refusing to collaborate with lay midwives. "You know," he said in a burst of candor, "the only reason the D.A. is going on this sort of case is that he's getting the screws put to him by the medical profession. Doctors don't want to see those midwives out there. They don't want someone stealing all their business."[41]

The chief of obstetrics at San Luis Obispo County Hospital, who had been a key figure for the prosecution, responded that he was "appalled" at Kilpatrick's statement and that the judge was speaking out of his jurisdiction. In his view, the case was clearly one of child abuse. As for the collaboration proposed by Kilpatrick, while he himself might tolerate working with a certified nurse midwife, his colleagues would not be so generous. They would allow a nurse midwife in one of their hospitals "over their dead bodies."[42]

The Santa Cruz case had resulted in what was essentially a draw between the midwives and the legal and medical forces opposing them. In San Luis Obispo, the acquittal of Doshi meant a clear-cut victory. In the third case which began in November 1979, when another California midwife delivered an apparently lifeless infant, the prosecution was determined to gain an unequivocal judgment against midwifery in general and Rosalie Tarpening in particular. In the process, she was subjected to some of the harshest treatment meted out to a modern-day midwife.

Tarpening, a licensed physical therapist in her early fifties, shared a practice with her chiropractor husband in Madera, a town in California's Central Valley. She had taken up midwifery in 1972 when women came to her asking for help, and she claimed that at the time she had checked with the district attorney's office about the legality of attending births at home and been told there was no law against it. As a self-educated naturopath and nutritionist, she was, until that November day, fairly confident of her ability to help women give birth safely, no matter what their initial condition. She was also a deeply religious woman who believed in the sanctity of the family and the significance of birth as a family event, and she had built up a following of grateful women.

Maternity cases accounted for about one-fifth of her practice.

She charged a fairly stiff fee (nine hundred dollars) for perinatal care that included nutrition and exercise advice and delivery, but seldom collected the entire amount, according to her bookkeeper.[43] In contrast, the obstetrical staff of the local community hospital charged sixteen hundred dollars per pregnancy and delivery. Furthermore, earlier that year they had directed the hospital to turn away any patient in labor (unless birth was imminent) who had not received prenatal care from one of them. Hispanic women frequently turned up at the hospital emergency room in the midst of labor, and the obstetricians were tired of having to attend women who had had no prenatal care. Yet, like most of their California colleagues, few Madera doctors would accept patients on Medi-Cal, the state medical assistance program. (As of 1977, only 37 percent of California obstetricians accepted Medi-Cal patients.) So the poor women of Madera and the surrounding communities were in a predicament when they considered where and how to deliver their babies. For many, a lay midwife was the only solution.

It was in this atmosphere that Graciella Villa, an undocumented alien, had come from Fresno seeking Tarpening's aid during pregnancy. The birth took place in Tarpening's home, something the midwife knew to be risky since local authorities had been aware of her practice by a stalled birth in 1977. That incident, resulting in a cesarean at the community hospital, dramatized the lay midwife's dilemma: if doctors refused to provide backup, she had no recourse but to take her clients to the emergency room where the reception, certainly in Madera, was likely to be hostile. When Gabriel Villa was born after a fairly easy labor but was clearly in trouble, Rosalie tried gentle resuscitation without result and then, following the only course open to her, sent her assistant with the baby to Madera Community Hospital. She herself stayed with the mother who had not yet delivered the placenta. In the emergency room, the infant was pronounced dead after resuscitation efforts failed. The autopsy report laid blame on Tarpening: "Baby died as a result of negligence on the part of the person who delivered it."[44]

On November 30, an armed posse accompanied by police photographers and a representative from the Bureau of Medical Quality Assurance showed up at the Tarpening home to arrest Rosalie on charges of murder, grand larceny, and four counts of practicing medicine without a license. She was held on one hundred thousand dollars bail and put in jail. A week later when bail was lowered to twenty-five thousand dollars, she and her husband mortgaged their home to post bond, and Rosalie was freed pending legal proceedings which dragged on for months. At the first hearing, prosecuting attorney Paul Avent appeared late and without witnesses, having forgotten the date. When the judge dismissed charges, Avent immediately rearrested Tarpening and took her off to jail where, once again, she was fingerprinted, stripsearched and incarcerated. Meantime sources of support were galvanized across the state and nation, including groups concerned with women's health and the right to give birth at home. One of the most active was NAPSAC.

The district attorney's office presented a picture of Tarpening as brutal and greedy. District Attorney David Minier, saying his information came from the coroner's report, told the press the baby's skull had been crushed during delivery. Paul Avent, whose vindictiveness against Tarpening never abated through the long months of hearings, said she was motivated only by desire for money. Tarpening's supporters did not allow such allegations to pass unchallenged: "Arise, citizens of Madera. Do not let the District Attorney make Madera the medical witch hunt capitol of the nation. He has charged Rosalie Tarpening with murder for assisting at the birth of a child that was stillborn. Such an absurd prosecution at the taxpayers' expense can only besmirch the very image of Madera."[45] So read a mailing sent out by Tarpening's defense committee, headed by David Peterson of Monterey.

During the year of pre-trial hearings, the longest in Madera County history, Tarpening was forced to listen silently to affirmations of the most serious charges against her offered by a stream of expert witnesses. One, the medical examiner and coroner of San Francisco, declared, "I believe that prompt and complete resuscitation of this baby would have delivered a normal child." Another, the head of obstetrics at a Fresno hospital, testified that in his opinion the infant had been born alive and capable of being saved.[46]

During the months that followed, while the defense, headed again by Anne Cumings, prepared to present its most valuable witness, Rosalie Tarpening saw her practice fall sharply. In November, nearly a year after the event, the defense presented a single witness in rebuttal, a tiny white-haired woman named Edith Potter. Then seventy-nine years old, she had been considered before her retirement one of the seven top pathologists in the world. Her major work, *Pathology of the Fetus and Infant*, had been cited previously by the prosecution witnesses. Dr. Potter was not in favor of home births or even of the practice of midwifery, as later correspondence showed, but she knew a botched autopsy when she saw one. A former professor at the University of Chicago Medical School, Potter said the autopsy performed on Gabriel Villa would have earned an *F* had one of her students done it. She charged the report with asserting as the cause of the baby's death two conditions commonly found in normal newborns: bleeding inside the skull, and the presence of amniotic fluid in the lungs which merely showed the infant had breathed while still in the uterus.

At the close of the morning's testimony, Potter startled everyone by saying that there was no doubt the baby had been born alive. This ran directly counter to the belief of Tarpening and her supporters that the baby was stillborn, and there was a buzz of fearful speculation over what this testimony would do to the defense. Early in the afternoon session, Potter banished those fears with an assessment of Gabriel Villa's death that electrified her audience. He had been brought to the Madera Hospital alive, she said, and capable of further resuscitation as shown by electrocardiograms. Three ECGs had indicated a normal heartbeat—the fourth electrocardiogram, made after the final vigorous resuscitation, showed a dying infant. The cause of death? The autopsy reports revealed the truth—the liver and diaphragm displaced, the stomach distended by air and both lungs filled with too much air at too great a pressure, pumped into the infant's lungs in an effort to force him to breath. "No baby can survive under these conditions. This baby was blown up."[47]

In the words of journalist Mark Hunter, the prosecuting attorney was "reduced to a straight man for the defense."[48] In response to his queries, attempting to show that an infant who was apparently not breathing could not survive without prompt resuscitation, Potter replied on the contrary, that such infants could survive indefinitely. She told the story of a seemingly lifeless baby born at the University of Chicago Medical Center who had been sent to the autopsy room where a doctor, lifting his knife for the first cut, saw the infant move an arm.

As a result of Dr. Potter's testimony, the murder charge was dismissed. However, the more provable charge remained, and Tarpening finally went to trial for practicing medicine without a license. Cumings felt she could probably not get an acquittal so she moved aside, making room for Gail Roy Fraties, an attorney who had worked on other home birth cases. In his own words, he was a "tough, mean trial lawyer," just the sort that midwives, who were usually kindly and trusting people, needed for defense in court. He had already successfully defended an Alaskan doctor, Peter Rosi, in a similar case and hoped to do the same for Tarpening.

On August 21, 1981, after two days of deliberation, Tarpening's jury pronounced her guilty of one misdemeanor count of practicing medicine without a license. Fraties asked for an acquittal. The probation officer proposed thirty months in jail to teach Tarpening respect for the law, and Avent argued that she should be fined thirty thousand dollars. Judge Clifford Plumley, himself born at home, made reference to Tarpening's fifty-five years of life without a blemish when he handed down judgment in September. His sentence, which provoked Avent to cries of "rape," was a one-year jail term, suspended, with the stipulation that she not attend any births for two years, even as a coach.

Although doctors connected with NAPSAC recommended that the emergency room staff be subjected to disciplinary proceedings for conspiring to hide the facts of Gabriel Villa's death, no action was taken, while Rosalie Tarpening, nearly broken after two years of accusation, uncertainty, and considerable financial loss, was free to return to what remained of her physical therapy practice without further fine or time in jail. She had suffered personally as well as professionally, in part from her own doubts about what she could have done to save the baby, and continued to suffer in the aftermath of the trial. When she appeared at a preliminary hearing for midwife Teri Calhoun in early 1982, Tarpening showed the effects of physical and emotional exhaustion from the long ordeal; still, she offered courage and support to the younger midwife who was also accused of murder.

Neither Calhoun's case nor subsequent others drew the media interest and fanfare that accompanied the earlier arrests.[49] Some activists believe this is the effect of a deliberate strategy to keep public support from building in favor of the midwives. In the absence of well-researched news stories defining the issues common to all midwife arrests, such as Mark Hunter's "Mothers and Outlaws" (*New West*, December 1980), the individual case was most easily seen as an isolated, if pitiful, event. NAPSAC's charge of a national conspiracy to eliminate all out-of-hospital practitioners could then be dismissed as nonsense.

But if the California arrests are viewed in the context of a stream of related cases across the country, a pattern emerges that tends to support NAPSAC's thesis. In 1979, Carolle Baya was repeatedly charged by the state of Florida for practicing medicine without a license, although she had applied for a midwife permit several times and been refused. (Unlike California, Florida had granny midwife laws still on its books.) In Illinois, Hope Valera Davis, a registered nurse trained in home birth techniques by a physician, was accused of violating the Nurse Practice Act. She organized sympathizers who subsequently filed a class action suit. They succeeded in overturning a statute that had discontinued issuance of midwife permits in 1965, but typically, when Davis was free to practice, she could not find a doctor willing to back her up. In New Mexico, midwife Tish Demmin was forced into a two-year fight with the state health agency over the reissuance of midwife permits. In Kansas and New Jersey, licensed nurse midwives took to the courts to secure more representation on state boards that were regulating them out of existence.

One of the best organized groups, the Association for Childbirth at Home (ACHI) had been under investigation since 1978 when the Illinois attorney general charged it with consumer fraud because ACHI refused to turn over its lists of childbirth educators and lay midwives. After Illinois subpoenaed seventy-three items from its files, ACHI appealed to the state supreme court. In 1981, Amanda Hess, a member of the U.S. Air Force, sought ACHI's help when she was threatened with court-martial and forced hospitalization if she persisted in having a baby at home with a midwife. The group, together with the American Civil Liberties Union, gathered evidence demonstrating that military hospitals in Hess's area had higher complication rates and administered more drugs than were usual in labor and delivery. This information was given to the press, and as a result of the publicity, the authorities allowed Hess to have her baby at home.[50]

These and other incidents of harassment continued to occur in the United States and Canada while medical societies quietly worked to eradicate competition. Not only were lay midwives targeted, but attempts to curtail nurse practitioners and nurse midwives were also apparent. In 1981 an Idaho physician alerted colleagues to the proliferation of non-physician health personnel. A copy of his speech was mailed to every state medical society and in some states to every physician. He warned that "doctors must maintain total power over all health care providers and any proposed legislation that would expand the practice scopes of nurses or others should be strongly opposed."[51] In June 1981, the AMA voted to oppose federal funding for training nurse practitioners and nurse midwives.[52]

## Aftermath of the Midwife Arrests

The exposure of birth practices brought about by widely publicized hearings generated some significant changes in health care for pregnant women. The aims of reformers were further encouraged by investigations of a photojournalist named Suzanne Arms. A young mother who had been radicalized by personal experience with the American way of birth, Arms published the results of her investigations in a book titled *Immaculate Deception* in 1975. In the first of what would become a series of published attacks on the health system as it affected women, the book, with its startling title, provided powerful support for charges made in other formats by Doris Haire and Lester Hazell. As Haire had done a few years earlier, Arms traveled to Holland and Denmark to view birth practices; back home she visited maternity wards and interviewed midwives, including Raven Lang, as well as doctors. She concluded that standard maternity care in the U.S. constituted a deception based on the conviction that hospitals were the only safe environment for a frightening and dangerous event, and doctors the only appropriate attendants. "The result is that birthing mothers have given up their responsibility in normal birth to obstetricians who have turned the normal into the abnormal . . . under the immaculate protection of the sterile hospital environment, the home of medical technology."[53]

As a result of such criticism, hospital administrators began to establish alternative birth centers in the hope of satisfying women who might otherwise seek out midwives and home births. Another outcome in California was that nurse midwives finally achieved the legal right to practice. A third, less concrete but possibly more influential, change in that state was the radical shift in attitude that followed the election of Jerry Brown as governor. So profound was this change that seven years after Walker, Bowland, and Bennett were carted off to jail to be booked for practicing medicine without a license, the Department of Consumer Affairs, the very agency chosen to bring them down for the sake of protecting the public, sponsored an important series of hearings on the current status of health care for all California woman and their newborns, in which midwives emerged as heroines instead of imposters.

Held during March and April 1981, in the urban centers of Oakland and Los Angeles, and in Fresno and Chico, two central California cities serving a surrounding rural population, the hearings were sponsored by a coalition of government agencies, legislators on the state and federal level, as well as representatives of consumer groups and racial and ethnic minorities. They provided a forum for the testimony of more than one hundred witnesses on what the DCA deemed a "deepening crisis in health care." A resulting four hundred-page report, published the following year, stands as a compendium of what childbirth reformers had been saying for the past thirty or forty years was wrong with the American way of birth and how it could be put right. Witnesses asserted that the existing system of perinatal care was inadequate, that poor women and children suffered from high death and complication rates far above those of the middle class, that healthy mothers often received high-technology obstetrical care that was both costly and of questionable benefit, while poor women who could have benefited from preventive services did not receive them. They also suggested that many infants saved by new techniques were permanently disabled and were sent home without vital follow-up support for them and their parents. Testifying as to the existence of these conditions, Professor Angela Davis said:

> As growing numbers of medically indigent women are forced to go without prenatal care and proper nutrition, thus producing very low birth weight babies, every effort is made to keep those infants alive . . . through the use of expensive, profit-making technology. . . . The medical establishment's . . . solution to an embarrassingly high rate of infant mortality in this country's poor and Third World communities is increased reliance on the technological miracles that keep low birth weight babies alive, many of whom are born prematurely because their mothers could not obtain early equal respectful care . . . [54]

In exploring the origin of such solutions to obstetrical care, the DCA report laid blame on a new and dangerous alliance: " . . . priorities in medical care are set by the medical industrial complex, which focusses on providing health care at a profit. Prevention, by definition, is not profitable except in terms of human life."[55]

Blame was also charged to the way in which doctors were trained, an education supported to a large extent by state and federal funding and, therefore, by taxpayers. According to one witness, the system limited students' contact almost exclusively to specialists and subspecialists in medicine, providing no introduction to other personnel whose training lay in prevention, such as nutritionists, midwives, and childbirth educators. The system imposed a rigid and exhausting schedule on novice physicians, in a process "more intense than in any other profession, with the possible exception of the military."[56] After a decade of such training, new doctors emerge with the conviction that they deserve the adulation that comes with an M.D. degree. In a newspaper feature questioning whether the admission of more women into medicine would humanize the profession, a journalist quoted his physician-wife: "It's difficult . . . to remember that you're actually a public servant. It's very hard to keep that in mind when all of society worships physicians and you have such enormous power."[57]

Student doctors also become highly skilled in the use of tools and equipment, while other areas of healing, particularly those concerned with nutrition, counseling, and basic preventive medicine, are almost totally ignored. This, the DCA noted, was particularly significant for obstetrician-gynecologists, most of whose future patients would be healthy women, whose training emphasized high-risk pregnancies and the use of very expensive technological tools without reference to the cost to the patients, either in dollars or well-being. Furthermore, increasing dependence on technology in both training and practice had produced the alliance between doctors and the producers of the equipment that now exercised enormous influence on health care. "This emphasis on treatment is rooted in the economic structure of the health services industry and in trends toward increased medical specialization and use of medical technology."[58]

Witnesses said the trend was particularly evident in the burgeoning use of neonatal intensive care units where newborns threatened by prematurity, low weight, or other conditions are placed for care at an astronomical cost. Although a recent development, "neonatal intensive care has already managed to equal or surpass the cost of some of the most expensive adult services, such as coronary bypass surgery and plastic surgery."[59] According to figures gathered at UCSF Medical Center in 1980, each infant that weighed less than one kilogram (2.2 pounds) cost an average of $46,340 to save.[60] And even if the infant survived the first critical days, it might well die later more slowly and more expensively. Costs in some such cases exceeded sixty thousand dollars. There were other disturbing questions about the new techniques which echoed those of reformists like Doris Haire. One study had found that approximately 30 percent of low birth weight infants have major handicaps.[61] Did the circumstances surrounding the use of neonatal technology play some part in creating additional long-term problems for critically ill newborns?

Focus on cost produced another consumer charge. A witness noted that maternity wards had traditionally been run at a loss in most hospitals. The innovation in new neonatal technologies, the use of which is reimbursed at very high rates by either insurance companies or the state or federal government, has turned perinatal care into one of the most profitable aspects of the hospital industry. And, as elsewhere, the expense is ultimately borne by the taxpayer.[62] Overall, the DCA report charged, the cost effectiveness of preventive care was five times greater than that of crisis treatment.[63]

The questions about neonatal technology affected minority groups particularly. In the black community, for example, the incidence of low birth weight infants has not declined, and proportionately, more black women die giving birth and more black babies die at birth or in the neonatal period. Just prior to the hearings, a Sacramento paper carried a story on the disturbing gap between the affluent and the poor in health care: "In the East Oakland black ghetto, the infant death rate is six times as high as in the nearby affluent Oakland Hills. . . . Although the maternal death rate has been sharply reduced, it is currently three times as high for blacks as for whites."[64]

DCA witnesses produced statistics showing similar conditions prevailed in other minority groups. In California, Hispanic women are further alienated on the basis of language differences and often on questions of legality of residence, although their infants will become citizens at birth. Evidence also showed that pregnant and delivering Asians and Native Americans were being neglected in the "deepening crisis in health care."

In the final report, the DCA endorsed a recommendation that California "actively promote nurse and non-nurse midwifery services as one means of providing cost-effective, comprehensive perinatal services which have been shown to be effective in lowering perinatal morbidity and mortality rates . . . "[65] In a complete reversal of its former stance, the department supported each of three bills aimed at providing licensure and regulation of lay midwives. After the defeat of the second bill, Michael Krisman, Chief Deputy Director of the DCA, sent a letter to supporters: "(In) four hours of testimony, the only opposition was from the California Medical Association and the local chapter of the American College of Obstetricians and Gynecologists. Both groups took the position that women should not have the option of a midwife-attended birth."[66] The third try encountered the same opposition and also failed. The AMA, having campaigned so successfully in the nineteenth century to outlaw competition, continued in the latter quarter of the twentieth to make certain the descendents of the old "irregulars" were kept out of the health field.

So lay midwives remained illegal in California, but nurse midwives had been licensed to practice in the state for seven years at the time of the hearings, where witnesses testified to the value of their services. Madeleine Shearer, editor of *Birth*, told the story of an experiment using nurse midwives in Madera County more than a decade before the profession was legal. "Three nurse midwives . . . went into the field . . . (and) began to bring in high-risk, malnourished, overworked farm worker women . . . (and) gave them prenatal care." Eventually the midwives were performing more than 60 percent of the deliveries and had doubled the number of women receiving prenatal care in the first trimester. During this time, premature births dropped from 11 percent to 6.4 percent, and neonatal deaths were halved from nearly 23.9 in every thousand births to only 10.3. "The major figure of 10/1,000 births (which) is the current goal of the American College of Obstetrician/Gynecologists . . . was reached twenty years ago in Madera among a very large, a very high risk population without any technology but with primary care."[67] Typically, when funding for the project ran out, it was terminated and the midwives sent away. Soon the incidence of prematurity and deaths among newborns in Madera began to climb again, the death rate later tripling to 32.1 per thousand. A study was made that demonstrated the loss of midwifery service was responsible for the increase in prematurity and neonatal deaths. Nevertheless, the lesson for the California health system was not taken seriously, and nurse midwives had to wait another eleven years before receiving legal status.[68]

Even after attaining licensure, their ability to practice was sharply limited, as the DCA hearings demonstrated. In California as elsewhere, three stumbling blocks made the practice of midwifery difficult even for the most determined. First, the nurse midwife had to find a hospital willing to grant her privileges; then she had to search for doctors willing to provide medical backup in the event of emergency. If she was lucky enough to get that far, she had to fight for reimbursement from Medi-Cal or other insurers, even when the charge for her services was decisively lower than that demanded and received by obstetricians in the area. The next likely occurrence was that the doctor who had contracted with her for back-up services, informed that his or her malpractice insurance had been quietly cancelled, revoked the contract with the midwife in order to regain insurance. Typically, the midwife then gave up and turned to friendlier territory—family planning clinics or public health.

The DCA saw other solutions: "All barriers should be aggressively addressed through negotiations and litigation where appropriate."[69] Following the replacement of Governor Brown with conservative George Deukmejian, in January of 1983, the state consumer and health agencies, who along with everyone else faced severe budget cuts, seemed much less likely to join such battles. But the message had not gone unheard. Litigation emerged in the eighties as a primary weapon for advocates of childbirth reform.

## Nashville Story

Litigation is what was used in Nashville, Tennessee, in a case in which the nurse midwives did not quietly go away but took to the courts in one of the first tests of whether professional medicine could retain its century-long control of all American health care. Two nurse midwives, Victoria Henderson and Susan Sizemore, had been practicing in the Maternal Infant Program at Metro Nashville General Hospital for five years. However, when they ventured to open a private practice (Nurse Midwifery Associates), trouble began. Three local hospitals whose medical staff by-laws permitted the practice of non-physician providers first delayed and eventually refused to grant the women staff privileges. Dr. W. Darrell Martin, who had contracted to provide medical backup for the midwifery service, was told that his malpractice coverage would not be renewed at the end of the year. The reason given by the physician-owned insurance company was that Martin's practice now involved "increased risk exposure of such proportions" that coverage could no longer be provided.[70] Threatened by rumors that his medical colleagues planned to ruin him professionally, Martin left Nashville with his family to practice medicine somewhere else. Henderson and Sizemore could not find any other doctor willing to take his place. The women concluded that they had been allowed to practice without harassment as long as they were dealing with poor and welfare patients in a clinic, but the threat of economic competition when middle-class women chose midwives over obstetricians fueled the campaign against Nurse Midwifery Associates.

In late 1980, the two midwives closed their program and transferred clients to other providers, but they had not entirely given up. Joined by Dr. Martin and a consumer couple, they filed a lawsuit in federal court, March 2, 1982, naming five doctors and three hospitals and the physician-owned insurance company in a charge of restraint of trade. The case scheduled to go to trial October 31, 1983, was postponed until summer 1984. In spite of the drain of energy and financial resources involved in waging a legal battle, the midwives held fast, encouraged by support from around the country and particularly from the American College of Nurse Midwives (ACNM). Their case was further validated by the decision of a federal district court in Nashville, in the fall of 1982, that the insurance company and its doctor-director were not immune from charges of boycott leading to a restraint of trade, as they had claimed.[71]

The basis of the Nashville suit in the antitrust provisions of the Federal Trade Commission raised the spectre of a small army of mid-level practitioners bringing suit on the same grounds and sent ripples of anxiety through the ranks of the AMA. Their response was to push for federal legislation exempting physicians, dentists, and other professionals licensed by the states from any FTC antitrust action. The AMA lobbyists, among the best-paid and most powerful in Washington, went to work persuading congressmen to vote their way. They were successful in the House in September 1982, but lost in the Senate in December. "The good guys won for once," said Jay Angoff, attorney for Ralph Nader's Congress Watch group, although he warned that the AMA would doubtless try again for the exemption.[72] Early the following year, the Supreme Court upheld the FTC's jurisdiction over professionals in a review of a Virginia case, and the way was cleared for the Nashville midwives to seek redress of grievance in the courts.

In 1983, in San Jose, California, a British-trained midwife named Liz Summerhayes who, like Henderson and Sizemore, had lost hospital privileges when she expanded into private practice, filed a complaint against the hospital and twenty-one doctors. In the same city, another nurse midwife, Harriet Palmer, who had served on the ASPO board of directors for six years, struggled with the multiple frustrations of trying to obtain hospital privileges and medical backup. Using multiple delaying tactics over a period of years, Stanford University Medical Center frustrated any possibility of obtaining privileges. During that time, Palmer, with the sponsorship of Family Planning Alternatives in San Jose, helped open a facility called Birth Home which served largely low-income women. Although Palmer's service was popular, the parent agency found it could not bear the high cost demanded by physicians kept on call nor the struggle over whether they would retain their insurance. In September 1982, the FPA board voted to close Birth Home because of the insurance problems, and Harriet Palmer went into private practice. Ironically, she had just then won the coveted privileges in one local hospital but without institutional backing could not make use of them.

Palmer was finally able to secure medical backup for a home birth service and, in league with other nurse midwives, persevered in conducting a practice under conditions that many nurse midwives would reject as too unstable. Since none of the women had hospital privileges, in event of emergency they would have to relinquish care of their patients at the emergency room door, much as a lay midwife would. The difference is that a backup doctor with some knowledge of the case would then take over.[73]

Physicians saw themselves as further threatened by other health care people who demanded the right to practice within the system. Already doctors felt besieged on one side by unreasonable demands of consumer fads, and on the other by the threat of malpractice suits instigated, as one physician put it, by greedy lawyers and furthered by judges and legislators who used to be greedy lawyers.[74] The editor of a newsletter for the American College of Obstetricians and Gynecologists issued a warning to his fellows: "If we are to avoid being done in by the malpractice problem we must reassert our control over the patient and insist that we exclusively make the decisions ... putting an end to the non-physician interference in this process."[75]

At a conference on obstetrical technology sponsored by Shearer's *Birth* and other groups early in 1983, some obstetricians spoke in voices tinged with gloomy paranoia of being forced to use whatever technology was required by the local medical community, regardless of its advisability in individual cases. Otherwise, in the event of legal action, they could be convicted by a single expert witness of having provided substandard care.[76] In the afternoon, a young civil rights lawyer used terms of warfare in counseling mid-level practitioners on how they might use litigation to break the medical monopoly on health care. Doctors and hospitals who lock out nurse midwives from hospitals, he declared, are liable to antitrust action. In his home state of Virginia, they are also open to suit based on interference with a contractual relationship. In addition to the straightforward antitrust and restraint of trade suits, he listed possible action on a secondary level, using what he called the tactics of guerrilla warfare: educating the judiciary, supporting new laws, seeking favorable opinions from state attorney generals, or learning how best to influence hospital boards to expand privileges to include nurse midwives and others pushing for a share in providing health care.[77]

It appeared to the childbirth reformers that the changes they sought might finally come about as a part of larger campaigns to retain humane principles in general and to create new ones for a technological age. While some reformers girded for court battles, others struggled to maintain pioneer alternative birthing services already in place.

## Birthing Centers In and Out of Hospital

Soon after the Santa Cruz bust, hospital birthing centers sprang up in California and elsewhere. By 1980, there were over three hundred alternative birth centers (ABCs) in the country, varying in services and philosophy of care. Most advertised a homelike setting, a minimum of intervention (no routine preps, IVs, or fetal monitors), and welcomed family members, including children and friends of the laboring woman. They offered consumers a pleasant blend of home and hospital with the safety of emergency equipment near at hand. There were other advantages to the ABCs: they educated doctors and nurses who otherwise would never see a natural birth proceed at its own pace; they provided a haven for nurse midwives who were free to offer the kind of continuous care their training prepared them for; and awareness of the services they provided frequently increased flexibility on an adjoining conventional ward as staffers became more committed to the normalcy of labor.

One of the first and most successful ABCs was the New Life Center, the obstetrical unit of Family Hospital in Milwaukee, Wisconsin, which included a nurse midwifery service and offered alternatives unavailable in other local hospitals. On the West Coast, San Francisco General Hospital offered nurse midwives and flexible care in its Alternative Birth Center under the directorship of Rosemary J. Mann. A study published in the *American Journal of Obstetrics and Gynecology* in 1981 of the first thousand births in this center demonstrated no difference in either death or complication rates between babies delivered by nurse midwives and those delivered by doctors. Although women with serious complications were excluded from the program, criteria for admittance were more liberal than in other in-hospital birth centers and allowed for the delivery of five sets of twins in those first thousand births.[78]

However, not all alternative birth centers were committed to family-centered ideals. It was more difficult to qualify for admission to some of the centers, according to one nurse, than to compete in the Olympics. Sociologist Raymond DeVries made a survey of hospital birthing centers and discovered that few women received the full benefits of giving birth outside the delivery room and that about a third were transferred ("risked out") during labor.[79] What was loudly proclaimed in the media, Dr. Gary Richwald, director of a home birth service in Los Angeles noted, was not available to most women. "They (the centers) come about only when there is a financial crush; when a combination of falling birth rates, increase in out-of-hospital births, increase in general maternity costs (take place), then an alternative birth room occurs, not for quality care, not for family centered obstetrical care, but in direct response to cost control and competition."[80]

Free standing birth centers, operating outside hospital walls, remained truer to the concepts of natural birth. By 1983 nearly eighty of these centers were operating in the United States. One of the first was inaugurated by Ruth Lubic, CNM, Director of the Maternity Center in New York City in 1975. After she declared her intention, there was an uproar on the Maternity Center board of medical directors, leading to some resignations. In spite of this response and an ensuing two-year war with Blue Cross of Greater New York, Lubic persisted. She wanted a low-cost facility where nurse midwives could function as they had been trained, and she was determined to provide a model to show how midwifery could work in a big city with middle-class clientele. Unlike many others who established in-hospital birthing centers with high hopes, Lubic knew she couldn't do what she wanted in the institution. The needs of student doctors for experience, she said, took precedence over a patient's wishes. If an intern or medical resident needed to perform a certain procedure to meet training requirements, he or she would do it regardless of how the procedure interrupted the normal flow of labor and stressed the mother. In addition, expensive technical equipment was imposed on normal as well as high risk labors because its purchase price had to be repaid. Thus, the only way to avoid high-tech obstetrics was to remove birth from the hospital.

This philosophy put the Childbearing Center into direct competition with New York physicians and maternity wards, constituting what one writer termed a mini-boycott of the system. Lubic's response was that if the Childbearing Center was a boycott, it was also an answer for parents impatient with the current situation. "Today's young people look at their parents, the prime movers in organizations like the International Childbirth Education Association, La Leche League, and the American Society for Psychoprophylaxis in Obstetrics, and observe that they worked for two decades to get change and instead received tokenism."[81]

The Childbearing Center containing two birth rooms, a kitchen, bathrooms, a lab, a family room, and utility and office space, was built in the basement of MCA's headquarters on East 92nd Street in Manhattan. Despite the fact that births were safe and satisfying for its clientele, Lubic continued to have to deal with fierce resistance to the Center and with unfavorable rumors that have "slowed progress (but) have not been critical to our functioning." In her view, freestanding birth centers are old answers to the contemporary problem of young parents refusing to come into hospitals. The center was born, and in her words, "will be born again and again as perceived needs arise."[82]

In contrast to Lubic's big-city birth center, activist Ina May Gaskin set up an elaborate maternal-child health service, consisting of eight midwives, nurses, two doctors, ambulances, a pediatric clinic, a prenatal clinic, and a laboratory in a commune in rural Tennessee. Perhaps because the people she and the other lay midwives serve were not likely to seek conventional medical services, Gaskin has not been plagued with the legal and administrative problems Lubic suffered with the Childbearing Center. Midwifery systems have historically flourished in out-of-the-way places where there are few doctors. In backwoods Tennessee, Gaskin's maternity service is regarded as an asset by the local physician who provides backup and consultation services.

A former English teacher, Gaskin became a lay midwife after traveling with her husband Stephen and other cultural dissidents from California to rural Tennessee where they established a spiritual community named The Farm. Much of Gaskin's philosophy on birthing arises from her belief in the use of spiritual energy which she fully described in *Spiritual Midwifery* (1978). The low-technology birthing system at The Farm involves midwives with backup provided by doctors who are right there or nearby. One thousand births at the Farm showed a 1.5 percent Cesarean rate and a 1 percent use of the electronic fetal monitor. Infant outcome was excellent. "We think," wrote Ina May, "it is significant that these results were accomplished by amateurs, who took the trouble to teach themselves a discipline with almost no use of the technology . . . "[83]

Psychologist Judith Levy took over a bankrupt birth center at a feminist clinic in Gainesville, Florida, a university town where doctors did not welcome the competition. In contrast to other freestanding centers, Birthplace grew out of the women's health movement and Dr Levy's work on abortion rights. In 1979, Levy and Billye Y. Avery traced the center's origins:

> Beginning in the 1940s, the childbirth education movement sought to soften and reform hospital birth practices, but never challenged the idea of the hospital as the legitimate place to have a baby. . . . (Birthplace) is an expression of our belief that we have the right to make decisions about our bodies and ourselves. Without the fundamental choice to decide whether or not to conceive or whether or not to terminate a pregnancy, all other rights are illusionary. . . . It is our belief that traditional obstetrics which places us on our backs, knocks us out for delivery . . . symbolizes and actualizes the role of women in this society as passive victims.[84]

Keeping a community birth center going is, for Levy as for Lubic, an enormous and never-ending task. Whereas Lubic, as a prominent health professional, sustains support from sympathizers within the field as well as from parents, Levy relies primarily upon feminist and consumer support outside of the health system. In contrast to these two centers stands one of the few remaining hospitals in the United States dedicated solely to maternity care—Booth in Philadelphia.

"If there is one expression that curls my toes, it is the one about 'I *let* fathers into the delivery room' from an obstetrician, or even worse, from a parent, 'He *let* me hold my baby' always said with gratitude. We should be far past this!" said one of Booth's founders at a NAPSAC conference in 1979.[85] A childbirth educator and certified nurse midwife, Ruth Wilf was convinced that parents could be given the kinds of birth they wanted in a hospital setting.

In the summer of 1971, Wilf and a sympathetic obstetrician, John Franklin, and others set up midwifery services for a sixteen to eighteen-bed hospital to be called Booth Maternity Center. Formerly an underused Salvation Army facility serving unwed mothers in the inner city of Philadelphia, Booth soon earned a reputation for friendly, flexible care that brought in middle-class women as well as the indigent teenagers it was originally designed to serve. With the help of Kitty Ernst of the New York City Maternity Center, Wilf and Franklin made Booth a model of consumer-oriented, family-centered, non-interventionist hospital care. Ruth saw her role as elucidating the Booth philosophy which was, most significantly, to offer a single standard of care to all patients: "The best we have goes to everyone, regardless of means." Asked some years later for a comment on the program at Booth, she said the most interesting aspect was that it worked. After ten years, during which she became so identified with the hospital that one woman addressed a letter to "Ruth Booth," Wilf moved on to a different sort of practice, as the first nurse midwife to be employed by a hospital in southern New Jersey. Prior to being hired by John F. Kennedy Memorial Hospital, Washington Township Division, she worked with a parent group called New Visions for three years in order to secure the legal, medical, and community support she needed. A vital woman whose enthusiasm is continually renewed, Wilf believes that changes in birthing practices will come about only when parents demand them.[86]

In 1981, Ruth Wilf visited Raven Lang in the mountains of Ben Lomond, California. The two women shared their vision of a midwife training program that would combine both the "head" material of nurse midwifery and the "heart" material of lay midwifery. They both saw the value of such a mingling, but Raven was still hesitant about entering the established health system, fearing that state-regulated licensing for lay midwives might lead to their control by physicians, or perhaps their elimination. Still tinged with the views of a separatist, Raven recalled the Public Health nurses coming to her mountain house in 1971 and demanding to see her qualifications. "I qualify myself," she had said, looking at them straight and unblinking. "I qualify myself by my interest and my experience."

To American midwives, Raven Lang has remained a mythmaker, a rebel who never wavered even when she was called an outlaw. After the sojourn in Canada, where she set up three birth services and trained numerous lay midwives, she returned to California to give birth herself. In this birth after so long an interval, she was to reap the harvest of a thousand other labors attended and recorded, and hold her own child at the moment of birth as she had held so many others.

In the spring of 1976, the Kinzies came home just in time for the event. Raven went through the first stages of labor sitting in a tub of hot water, warm at last after the bitter winter on Vancouver Island. When the baby was about to be born, she moved from tub to bed, with her friend from the Birth Center, Kitti Lokas, as attending midwife. The friendly faces around Raven and the ferns and rough-hewn redwood walls receded from her consciousness. She felt she had descended beneath the world into interior chambers where she and Ken existed in perfect and protected solitude. After very little effort and far too soon for Raven, the baby was born. She reached down to feel between its legs to see if it was the girl she had wanted. Assured that it was, she fell into a state of bliss so intense that when Kitti told her she was "bleeding like a river," she didn't answer, but put the baby to breast in the time-honored manner and rapidly recovered as her uterus hardened.

The family had been given an abandoned chicken house at the foot of the orchard where Raven had taken her name. She and Ken transformed the tumble-down building into an artists' dwelling with bold paintings on the walls, Raven's loom in the corner, and sunlight streaming through skylights. Raven set up a weaving shop and attended only a few births for people in what she called her tribe, an extended family of like-minded friends. While she breastfed her daughter, Shaddah, she retreated from public life and enlarged her studies of birth to include the mysteries of spiritual healing. Like Ina May Gaskin who utilized the concept of energy fields in labor, Raven believed that emotion and energy could alter the course of a birth. She had seen that a calm presence could quicken labor and ease pain, and she had observed that maternity was a transformational process. She read about past cultures whose members held healing rituals to help people going through transformations of birth, puberty, marriage and death, ceremonies that appeared to aid those moving into another phase. The Blessing Way, a female puberty rite of the Navajos, held special significance for her and in time became her spiritual truth.

She began teaching poems, songs and chants that she had gathered for the Blessing Way at the Institute of Feminine Arts, a school designed to teach womanly skills and attitudes to those who wanted to become midwives. By supporting skills traditionally the province of women, the Institute teachers hoped to provide a counterforce in a society saturated with patriarchal myths and images.

These and other ideals were brought to a gathering of midwives in New Mexico in 1980 organized by Rajima Baldwin, the author of *Special Delivery* and president of the Informed Homebirth organization.[87] Among the midwives was the ailing Shari Daniels, Director of the El Paso Birth Center, who had shared her remarkable physical skill in complicated birth with many others. Under Raven's leadership, the women honored Shari with a Blessing Way. The seriously ill woman lay adorned with flowers while Raven washed her feet with sand and the others came to pay tribute and offer gifts. Then they danced and sang, not only in hope of sending healing energy to Shari Daniels, but to receive it themselves, healing the injuries of harassment and fear they all knew as midwives. Thus Raven brought an ancient ceremony into the midst of a modern struggle in the hope that the old ways of women's community would strengthen midwives under fire again in the twentieth century.

# CONCLUSION

Today we can be defeated in regard to laws, to appropriations, to representation, but if we are truly transforming consciousness, we cannot be defeated.

*Gerda Lerner.*[1]

In our journey through the lives of seven women and more than forty years of childbirth reform, we kept stumbling over a singular fact: what people call Lamaze, or "family centered maternity care," or a "Leboyer birth," are all aspects of skilled midwifery ideals that have always remained outside crisis-oriented medical care. Although Margaret, Elisabeth, Lester, Niles, Doris, Sheila and Raven would no doubt offer a variety of responses to questions of licensing, regulation and physical place allotted to birth, they have all at one time or another come to the same conclusion. And wasn't that what we all wanted to have: women attending women as they had done since the beginning of time? If so, how were reformers to resurrect a profession that had been thoroughly vilified and very nearly legislated out of existence?

As we discovered while working on Chapter Five, American midwifery has survived only in a sort of half-life, out of sight among the rural poor. Occasionally a pilot program like the one in Madera popped up, or notice was taken of a rare continuing service like the FNS in Kentucky, or a lone advocate called for revival. For the most part, however, reformers concentrated on effecting changes in the institutions we had all come to accept as inevitable, if not wholly beneficent.

Midwives began to resurface, we discovered, when reformers awoke to the suspicion that their chances of truly altering birth practices in hospitals where doctors remained in charge were not as rosy as originally supposed. In the beginning, it was assumed that doctors would eventually be persuaded, as Elisabeth Bing put it, "that normal labor does not occur only in retrospect." It was assumed that sooner or later they would accept the premise behind Doris Haire's advice on replacing fetal monitors with ironing boards, and would see the wisdom of keeping their hands in their pockets during normal labor, to use Sheila Kitzinger's phrase.

These assumptions continued to appear reasonable throughout the sixties and into the seventies. After all, the concept of a prepared birth was becoming widely known, at least among middle-class women, and childbirth education had grown from islands of influence like that produced by Margaret Gamper's work in the forties to a proliferation of classes offered all across the country. Furthermore, some remarkable goals had been achieved, many of them due to the efforts of the women featured in this book. The FDA withdrew approval of the elective use of oxytocin. Totally drugged labors were abandoned, and dosages of nearly all drugs were reduced. Breastmilk was finally recognized by the experts as superior to artificial formula. The concept of early mother-infant contact was accepted so completely that it became routine in many delivery rooms and the theory, if not the practice, of family-centered maternity gained a good deal of currency.

However, as Elisabeth Bing noted, all these accomplishments did not mean that the reformers had really gotten their way. By the end of the seventies, many educators saw that nearly every gain could be compromised if not actually swept aside by a wave of technological advance that served to strengthen existing institutions. In fact, childbirth in America in the eighties seemed likely to become a high-tech ritual beyond the control of nearly all birthing women. Some reformers despaired of ever prevailing against the specialty of obstetrics-gynecology which seemed, in Norma Swenson's words, to have "interpreted its mandate to define and control women's reproductive functions, a mandate endorsed not only by government, but by the people as well . . . "[2]

Most pregnant women still perceive their obstetricians as all-knowing in matters of childbirth, and most doctors share that view of themselves. Medical students are not selected for qualities which would allow future obstetricians to keep their hands in their pockets or wait patiently during labor, "watching a hole," as one put it long ago.[3] Nor does their subsequent experience encourage such qualities. Although the limitations of medical education are beginning to be recognized, there is little hope that the present generation of obstetricians (always with notable exception) will be readily persuaded to share power with their patients.

Even the long-sought goal of altering birth practice by bringing more women into the field now appears to have been misdirected. As Michelle Harrison demonstrated in the story of her experience as an obstetric resident, training in the speciality concentrates on interference, and the greatest satisfactions come from interfering successfully.[4] Women physicians (18 percent overall; 3.5 percent in obstetrics) are under enormous pressure to follow the prevailing ethic if they want to succeed.[5] Very few have been willing to risk their careers as ICEA pioneer Dr. Carolyn Mann Rawlins did over thirty years ago when she began offering instruction for family-centered deliveries in her Indiana practice. Several times, as a consequence of refusing to apply unnecessary intervention during labor, she had her hospital privileges revoked, a punishment that needs only to be threatened to bring the majority of obstetricians into line.[6]

One powerful element working against childbirth reform is the health industry, currently the fastest growing in the United States with profits accounting for more than ten percent of the GNP. Manufacturers have a vested interest in birth practices that require an array of costly machinery, and connections between the industry and the profession, like those between the military and manufacturers of weaponry, have produced a formidable alliance with the power to influence national policies. The partnership is further supported by a medical insurance system that rewards the use of costly technology and surgical intervention and penalizes those who choose more conservative methods. Government becomes part of the alliance when, bypassing the public, it relies solely on advice and information from the physicians and industrialists who stand to benefit economically and professionally from its decisions.[7]

In terms of birth care, the pregnant and delivering mother finds herself woefully ill-prepared for an encounter with this alliance of physicians, industrialists, and government agencies. Recently several independent sociological studies (Shaw, Scully, Oakley, and Rothman) demonstrated that the indoctrination which produces girls and women who see themselves as passive consumers in the health game still functions very well.[8] Even bolstered by consumer advocates like Lester Hazell and by La Leche League International and ICEA, few women find the courage to defy or even question their physicians, and seldom complain except to friends about disappointing hospital experiences. As Niles Newton concluded nearly thirty years ago, feminine passivity and dependence are traits opposite to those needed for good mothering, yet they are the ones given cultural approval. Few women are able to perceive with Adrienne Rich the blindness implicit in a society governed by patriarchal views:

> The woman awaiting her period or the onset of labor, the woman lying on a table undergoing abortion or pushing a baby out, the woman inserting a diaphragm or swallowing her daily pill, is doing these things under the influences of centuries of imprinting. Her choices, when she has any, are made or outlawed within the context of laws and professional codes, religious sanctions, and ethnic traditions, from whose creation women have historically been excluded.[9]

Of those few who do raise their voices, fewer still remain active in reform movements after their own childbirth experiences are past. For the rest, "faith in science and 'progress' is still too strong, (and) the sense of isolation and vulnerability is too powerful."[10]

Given the opposition of major institutions and the compliance of many women, how can we expect to revive the discredited midwife, an even more vulnerable target than reformers working to change the system from within? In California, for example, any midwife who comes to the attention of the authorities finds herself engaged in a struggle with the powerful medical lobby, a group that donates more money to political candidates than any other political action group in the state.[11] Equally lopsided contests are being acted out elsewhere whenever organized medicine defends its position as the only legitimate purveyor of maternity care.

Still, in the face of what seems a very unequal struggle, there is reason to believe that time may be on the side of the midwives — Daughters of Time as they often call themselves. Aside from the effect of agitation for reform, the major causes of optimism are the popular concern with wellness and the worry over escalating medical and hospital costs, both of which favor an expansion of alternative practitioners. Recently, in what might be viewed as a small Popular Health Renaissance, homeopath Dana Ullman and supporters, including Suzanne Arms who believed that midwives could be helped by the campaign, called on the California Board of Medical Quality Assurance (BMQA), armed with official statistics and demanding licensing for qualified lay practitioners.

Supporting his claim with impressive evidence, Ullman testified that safe alternatives can in some cases be more beneficial than costly medical treatments, that medical procedures in common usage work only ten to twenty percent of the time, and that although one out of eight prescription drugs has been shown ineffectual, doctors continue to prescribe them.[12] Surprisingly, one BMQA medical man responded, "There's plenty of evidence that people . . . have been helped by approaches most M.D.s are unable or unwilling to consider."[13] If Ullman's effort succeeds, and he sees it as a long-term struggle, it will unlock a door closed since the end of the nineteenth century to anyone except allopathic medical practitioners. Clearly related to the California uprising are other legal battles of the eighties: the nurse midwife cases in Nashville and San Jose covered in Chapter Five; four chiropractor-association suits against the AMA; and the recent outlawing of the pregnancy drug bendectin, partially as a result of pressure by women's health groups.

Probably an even more powerful incentive for change is the urgent need to reduce the inflation in health costs—running at 18 percent in 1983 in contrast to about 4 percent for the general cost of living.[14] Taxpayers must continue to cover these skyrocketing bills for a swelling group of elderly, disabled, and unemployed Americans. In terms of value for money, midwives, along with other mid-level practitioners, begin to look better and better. Already the United States Army and Air Force have integrated nurse midwives into military hospitals where physicians are learning to accept them as colleagues. In another move for economy, Mayo Clinic is now housing medical patients undergoing expensive tests at a nearby motel instead of in the hospital.[15] Thus, in bits and pieces, precedents are broken and trends set that support female practitioners and out-of-hospital services. In another decade, it is not inconceivable that independent birth centers, like the maternity motel proposed by Lester Hazell in the sixties, will be accepted health care settings.

Another force favoring a return of midwifery is the women's health movement which has brought about many significant changes. As a result of feminist activism, more women are able to plan their children; more have a positive image of themselves and their bodies, and more are aware of their rights in a medical situation. To cite specific examples, fewer women will sign what used to be routine permission for the entire breast to be removed while the woman was still on the operating table for a biopsy and, thanks in good part to the work of Rose Kushner, most breast cancer victims are also aware of alternatives to radical surgery.[16] Other women facing potential disease brought about by hormones given to their mothers are able to find support in feminist DES action groups.

Although not always acknowledged, there are strong links between the women's health movement and childbirth organizations. Both groups attempt to change existing health services; both create alternatives to provide care consistent with their ideals (as in feminist women's clinics and freestanding birth centers) and both use the process of consciousness raising to increase self-esteem and confidence. Many women have moved from one cause to the other. Norma Swenson, an activist we have quoted at length, entered the reform movement as a member of the International Childbirth Education Association. After completing a term as president in 1968, she moved on to work with a group of women in Boston who were engaged in writing a pamphlet on women's health. The pamphlet grew into the very influential *Our Bodies, Our Selves* which has helped thousands of women to "understand, accept, and be responsible for (their) physical selves."[17]

While many women come into childbirth education classes motivated by the ideals of the women's movement, others come out of frustration over disappointing birth experiences. In 1983, Gay Courter addressed the American College of Nurse Midwives on the use of anger as a catalyst for change, saying she herself was moved by anger when she was writing her novel, *The Midwife*. Afterwards many readers wrote in response to a scene in which the heroine gives birth in a hospital:

> Each wrote that the gruesome birth reminded them of their own experiences . . . this is precisely the reaction I wanted . . . I wanted women to use anger . . . to review the way we give birth . . . When you get angry with physicians who . . . protect their power . . . angry at the way midwives are treated . . . turn these negative emotions into a vehicle for change.[18]

Fueled by anger or not, there is good evidence of the midwives' growing strength in their new willingness to seek unity among themselves. In the mid-seventies, David and Lee Stewart encouraged unification by their practice of putting lay and nurse midwives on the same podium at NAPSAC conferences. Following this precedent, Sister Angela Murdough, President of the American College of Nurse Midwives, invited leaders from the lay and licensed ranks to talk to one another in Washington in 1981. Of this precedent-breaking meeting, Genna Withrow wrote in the NAPSAC News, that the midwives met "as equals in a profession. We realized how time and maturity has led us to the point where we could recognize each other as valuable assets, not only for the community of families we serve, but for each other as well . . . The time has come . . . for an organization that can represent the ideals of midwifery in America."[19]

The Midwives Association of North America (MANA) was formed

on the spot and in 1983 held an organizational meeting in Colorado. There Amish, Mexican, Mormon, and Hassidic women, emerging from cultural confinement, made common cause with the others: feminists determined above all that women should have control of their reproductive powers; traditionalists intent on preserving the integrity of the family; midwives campaigning for licensing; others who, like Raven Lang, asserted women's right to qualify themselves— all bound together as women who attended other women in birth.[20] This show of solidarity, including women traditionally isolated, seemed certain to have a strong influence on the group and through it on the greater community. As Elizabeth Davis has written, "A strong motive for becoming a midwife is the common desire of women to come closer to one another—not just emotionally as friends but in the powerful sense of working together and establishing support systems for one another."[21]

There is hope that unity among the midwives will spread to other women in a network of support with goals that move beyond childbirth to the larger world. It may not be too grandiose to envision with Ehrenreich and English that the awakening consciousness of women, aware of their connections with one another and with a yet unknown history, will help to bring about fundamental changes, moving toward "a society organized around human needs; a society in which childraising is not dismissed as each woman's individual problem but in which the nurturance and well-being of all children is a transcendent public priority."[22]

These are values widely shared by the midwives whose reappearance fills us with hope for the future. A midwife standing before the birthing woman, waiting to catch new life, represents more than herself in an act of attendance. Drawing us with her as witnesses to birth, free of the shields of machinery and institutional ritual, she helps remind us of our common origins and of the ways in which we recognize one another as human.

# NOTES

## INTRODUCTION

1. Norma Swenson, "Response," *Birth Control and Controlling Birth*, edited by Helen B. Holmes et al., (Clifton, N.J., Humana Press, 1980), p. 261.
2. Lester Hazell, interview with authors, 1979.
3. Quoted in Catherine R. Stimson, "Gerda Lerner and the Future of Our Past," *Ms.*, September 1981, p. 94.
4. Adrienne Rich, *Of Woman Born* (New York, Bantam, 1977), p. XIX.

## CHAPTER ONE

1. William L. Laurence, "Doctors Assail Twilight Sleep," *The New York Times*, May 15, 1936, p. 1.
2. Ibid.
3. Ibid.
4. Ibid.
5. Letters to the editor, *The New York Times*, May 18–19, 1936.
6. "Medieval Thinking About Childbirth," Editors, *Ladies' Home Journal*, October 1936, p. 4.
7. Editorial, *Nation*, June 3, 1936, p. 699.
8. Letters to the editor, *Nation*, July 25, 1936, pp 111–112.
9. Gena Corea, *The Hidden Malpractice* (New York, William Morrow, 1977), pp. 185–186.
10. Ibid., p. 188.
11. Harold Speert, *Obstetrics and Gynecology in America: A History* (One East Wacker Drive, Chicago, American College of Obstetricians and Gynecologists, 1979), pp. 187–188.
12. Frederick Leboyer, *Birth Without Violence* (New York, Alfred Knopf, 1980), pp. 26–27.
13. Quoted in Richard W. Wertz and Dorothy C. Wertz, *Lying-In: A History of Childbirth in America* (New York, Schocken, 1978), pp. 142–143.
14. Ibid, p. 143.
15. Paul De Kruif, "Why Should Mothers Die?," *Ladies' Home Journal*, March 1936, p. 9.
16. Quoted in Wertz & Wertz, *Lying-In*, op. cit., p. 122, from Charles Meigs, *Obstetrics*, (Philadelphia, 1852), p. 631.
17. Paul De Kruif, *Ladies' Home Journal*, June 1936, p. 100.
18. Paul De Kruif, *Ladies' Home Journal*, March 1936, p. 8.
19. Giovanna Breu, Interview with Beatrice Tucker, *Life*, August 18, 1972, p. 58.
20. Beatrice Tucker, autobiographical sketch, unpublished, Margaret Gamper's library, Glenview, IL, 1973.
21. Joseph B. DeLee, *Principles and Practices of Obstetrics* (Philadelphia, W. B. Saunders Co., 1913), p. XIII.

22. Quoted in Rebecca Rowe Parfitt, *Birth Primer* (Philadelphia, Running Press, 1977), pp. 116–118.
23. Ibid. p. 168.
24. Speert, op. cit., pp. 107–108.
25. Mary Breckenridge, "Maternity in the Mountains," *North American Review*, Volume 226, December 1928, pp. 765–768.
26. Eunice Ernst, "Fifty-Three Years of Home Birth Experience at the Frontier Nursing Service, Kentucky 1925–78," *Compulsory Hospitalization or Freedom of Choice in Childbirth*, Volume 2, edited by David and Lee Stewart (P.O. Box 428, Marble Hill, MO 63764, NAPSAC Publications, 1979), p. 505.
27. Ibid., p. 516.
28. *Log 1915–1980*, New York, Maternity Center Association, pp. 7, 12.
29. Ibid., p. 14.
30. Mary Ries Melendy, *Sex-Life, Love, Marriage* (Eugenic Publication Office, 633 Plymouth Place, Chicago, Ill., 1913), p. 403.
31. Grantly Dick-Read, *Childbirth Without Fear*, 4th edition, revised by Helen Wessel and Harlan F. Ellis M.D. (New York, Harper and Rowe, 1972), p. 272.
32. Ibid., p. 306.
33. De Kruif, op. cit., March, 1936, p. 101.
34. Quoted in Grantly Dick-Read, op. cit., p. 292.
35. J. C. Furnas, "What Price Pain?" *Ladies' Home Journal*, February, 1940, p. 24.
36. Lawrence Galton, "Motherhood Without Misery," *Colliers*, November 16, 1946, p. 13.
37. *Chicago Daily News*, May 2, 1949, p. 17 and *Chicago Herald American*, October 23, 1949, p. 8.
38. Margaret Gamper, *Preparation for the Heirminded* (Hammond, Ind., Sheffield, 1971), p. 15, available from Midwest Parentcraft Center, 627 Beaver Road, Glenview, IL, 60025.
39. Ibid., p. 61.
40. Margaret Gamper, *Heirminded News*, Winter, 1980, p. 10.

## CHAPTER TWO

1. Quoted in Richard W. Wertz and Dorothy C. Wertz *Lying-In A History of Childbirth in America* (New York, Schocken, 1979), p. 182.
2. Henry B. Safford, M.D., "Tell Me, Doctor," *Ladies' Home Journal*, February 1951, pp. 31, 160–161.
3. Joseph B. DeLee, M.D., *Obstetrics for Nurses* (Philadelphia, W. B. Saunders, 1916), p. 114.
4. Safford, op. cit.
5. Lester Hazell, personal communication, 1979.
6. Mary Lempke, letter to Margot Edwards, October 19, 1983.
7. Herbert Thoms, M.D., "The Challenge to American Obstetrics," *Ladies' Home Journal*, April 1960, pp. 81–115.
8. Interview with authors, February 1983.
9. Quoted in Rhondda Hartman, *Exercises for True Natural Childbirth* (New York, Harper & Row, 1975), pp. IX–XI.
10. Quoted in Coleman Romalis, "Taking Care of the Little Woman," *Childbirth:*

Alternatives to Medical Control edited by Shelly Romalis, (Austin, University of Texas Press, 1981), p. 102.

11. Elisabeth Bing, "Childbirth at Forty: Elisabeth Bing's Own Story," *Parents*, January 1980. pp. 96–97.

12. "Natural or Unnatural?," *Time*, January 19, 1953, p. 52.

13. Waldo L. Fielding, M.D., and Lois Benjamin, "The Medical Case Against Natural Childbirth," *McCalls*, June 1962, p. 185.

14. Edward A. Graber, M.D., "Natural or Unnatural?" *Newsweek*, March 15, 1965, p. 97A.

15. Graber, Ibid.

16. Monica Furlong, "Unnatural Childbirth," *Mademoiselle*, March 1962, p. 147.

17. Marjorie Karmel, *Thank You, Dr. Lamaze* (Garden City, N.Y., Doubleday, Dolphin Edition 1965), p. 31.

18. Fernand Lamaze, M.D., *Painless Childbirth* (New York, Pocket Books, 1972), p. 12.

19. Ibid, pp. 13–14.

20. *New York Times*, January 9, 1956, p. 1.

21. Karmel, op. cit., p. 94.

22. Ibid., pp. 101–103.

23. Ibid., p. 118.

24. Ibid., p. 149.

25. Ibid., p. 165.

26. Ibid., p. 133.

27. Marjorie Karmel, "A New Method of Painless Childbirth," *Harper's Bazaar*, June 1957, pp. 72 and 120.

28. Elisabeth Bing, *Six Practical Lessons for Easier Childbirth*, (New York, Bantam Edition 1969), p. 111.

29. Elisabeth Bing, *Having a Baby After Thirty* (New York, Bantam, 1980), pp. 156–9.

30. Ibid., pp. 161–162.

31. Elly Rakowitz, "ASPO: Birth and Growth of an Ideal," *The Mother's Manual*, January–February 1978, p. 31.

32. *The New York Times*, July 1, 1954, p. 29.

33. Ashley Montagu, "Babies Should be Born at Home," *Ladies' Home Journal*, August 1955, p. 85.

34. *Ladies' Home Journal*, Letters, October 1955, p. 8.

35. Sloan Wilson, "The American Way of Birth," *Harper's*, July 1964, p. 51.

36. Ibid., p. 54.

37. Letters, *Harper's*, September 1964, p. 6.

38. Gladys Denny Schultz, "Cruelty in the Maternity Wards," *Ladies' Home Journal*, May 1958, pp. 151–155.

39. Schultz, "Cruelty," *Ladies' Home Journal*, December 1958, p. 59.

40. Schultz, "Cruelty," *Ladies' Home Journal*, May, 1958, p. 154.

41. Ibid., p. 155.

42. Schultz, "Cruelty," *Ladies' Home Journal*, December 1958, p. 58.

43. Lester Hazell, *Commonsense Childbirth* (New York, G. P. Putnam's Sons, 1969), p. xx.

44. Margaret Hickey, "Training for Childbirth," *Ladies' Home Journal*, May 1953, p. 146.

45. Lester Hazell, *Commonsense Childbirth* (New York, Berkley Press, 1976), p. xxxii.

46. Hazell, Ibid., pp. 221–222.

47. Lester Hazell, ICEA conference, St. Petersburg, Florida, May 1974.

# CHAPTER THREE

1. Dana Raphael, *The Tender Gift: Breastfeeding* (New York, Prentice-Hall, 1973), pp. 47–48.
2. Quoted in P. E. Hartmann et al., "Breastfeeding and Reproduction in Women in Australia—A Review," *Birth and the Family Journal*, 8:4 1981, p. 215.
3. Judith Wertman, "New Views on Feeding Babies," *The Medical Forum*, August 1982, p. 3.
4. Frank Howard Richardson, "Breast Feeding: Going or Coming? And Why?" *Child-Family Digest*, May/June 1960, pp. 3–4.
5. Jane Addams quoted in Gail Rempert and Eugene Dermody, *Women Who Fought: An American History* (Cerritos College, 11110 Alonda Bl., Norwalk, CA 1981), p. 186.
6. Richardson, op. cit., p. 4.
7. Wallace B. Hamilton, "This is the Danger Month for Your Baby," *The Delineator*, July 1913, p. 7.
8. Ibid.
9. "Nestlé's Food, A Perfect Nutrient for Infants, Children, and Invalids," *The Delineator*, July 1913, p. 50.
10. "The Boycott Continues," *Birthing*, June 1980, p. 1.
11. Stephen Solomon, *The New York Times*, Section IV, December 6, 1981, p. 92.
12. Ibid.
13. *Birthing*, op. cit., p. 1.
14. Solomon, op. cit., p. 92. For another view of the Infact controversy, see *The Lactation Review*, Volume IV, no. 1, 1979 and Volume VI, No. 1, 1982, edited by Dana Raphael (666 Sturges Highway, Westport, Conn. 06880) Anthropologist Raphael conducted research in the Third World that showed most mothers practiced mixed feeding, supplementing their breastfed babies as a cultural practice rather than as influenced by the formula manufacturers. She and other scientists claim that infants older than three months cannot thrive on human milk alone in these nations.
15. *The New York Times*, June 6, 1981, p. 4.
16. Quoted in *Childbirth Without Pain Education Association Newsletter*, July 1982, p. 8.
17. Ibid.
18. Angela Glover Blackwell and Lois Salisbury, "Administrative Petition to Relieve the Health Hazards of Promotion of Infant Formula in the U.S.," *Birth and the Family Journal* op. cit., pp. 287–296.
19. Barbara Ehrenreich and Dierdre English, *For Her Own Good* (Garden City, NY, Anchor/Doubleday, 1978), pp. 62–64.
20. Quoted in Hartmann, op. cit., pp. 215–216.
21. Ashley Montagu, *Touching* (New York, Harper, 1971), p. 94.
22. Sister Marian Adrian, *La Leche News*, Jan/Feb 1963, p. 1.
23. Richardson, op. cit., p. 4.
24. Linda Blachman, "Dancing in the Dark," *Birth and the Family Journal*, op. cit., p. 275.
25. Raphael, op. cit., p. 57.
26. Michael Newton and Niles Rumely Newton "The Let-Down Reflex in Human Lactation," Reprinted from *Journal of Pediatrics* 33:6, 1948, p. 2.
27. Ibid., p. 2.
28. Ibid., p. 7.
29. Niles Newton, *Maternal Emotions* (New York, Paul Hoeber, 1955), p. 45.
30. Profile of Niles Newton, *Psychology Today*, July 1972, p. 6.

31. Niles Newton, "The Trebly Sensuous Woman," *Psychology Today*, July 1972, p. 71.
32. Ibid., pp. 68–69.
33. Newton, *Maternal Emotions*, op. cit., p. 92.
34. Niles Newton, "Childbirth Under Unusually Fortunate Circumstances," *Child-Family Digest* September 1953, p. 40.
35. Ibid., p. 45.
36. Niles Newton, "Charlotte Aiken: Grandmother of ICEA," *ICEA News*, Fall 1977, p. 1.
37. Niles Newton et al., "Parturient Mice: Effects of Environment on Labor," *Science*, Volume 151, 1966, pp. 1560–1561. See also Niles Newton et al., "Experimental Inhibition of Labor Through Environmental Disturbance," *Obstetrics and Gynecology*, Volume 27, 1966, pp. 271–277; and Niles Newton et al., "The Effects of Disturbance on Labor: An Experiment Using One Hundred Mice with Dated Pregnancies," *American Journal of Obstetrics and Gynecology*, Volume 101, 1968, pp. 1096–1102.
38. Niles Newton, "The Point of View of the Consumer," *Proceedings of the National Congress on the Quality of Life*, (Chicago American Medical Association, 1974,), p. 92.
39. Ibid., pp. 93–96.
40. Niles Newton, "Overview of the Social, Psychological, and Research Issues in the Psychology of Hysterectomy," *Emotion and Reproduction*, (Proceedings of the Fifth International Congress of Psychosomatic Obstetrics and Gynecology, Rome, 1977).
41. Diana Scully, *Men Who Control Women's Health* (New York, Schocken, 1980), p. 24.
42. 42. Michelle Harrison, "Birth as the First Experience of Mothering," *20th Century Obstetrics Now*, Volume 2, edited by David and Lee Stewart, (P.O. Box 428, Marble Hill, Mo 63764, NAPSAC Publications, 1977), pp. 585–587.
43. Niles Newton, "Breast Feeding," *Child-Family Digest*, October 1953, p. 72.
44. Niles Newton, "New Help for Nursing Mothers," *Child-Family Digest*, Sept/Oct 1960, p. 45, 48.
45. La Leche League International, Inc., *La Leche League Love Story* (9616 Minneapolis Ave., Franklin Park, Illinois, 1978), p. 4.
46. Barbara Katz Rothman, *In Labor: Women and Power in the Birthplace*, (New York, Norton, 1982), pp. 204–205.
47. *La Leche League Love Story*, op. cit., p. 47.
48. Letter to Margot Edwards, August 18, 1980, p. 1.
49. Letter, *La Leche League News* 17:4, 1975, pp. 50–51.
50. Betty Wagner, *La Leche League News* 8:5, 1966, p. 5.
51. Quoted in Edwina Froelich, "Can LLL Be 20 Years Old?" *La Leche League News* 18:4, 1976, p. 1.
52. Ibid., p. 1.
53. Telephone interview with Margot Edwards, 1978.
54. Telephone interview with Margot Edwards, 1980.
55. Barbara Popper and Betty Ann Countryman, LLLI Information Sheet #80, La Leche League International, Inc. Franklin Park, Illinois.
56. Rothman, op. cit., p. 108.
57. Quoted in Blachman, op. cit., p. 271.
58. Quoted in "A Psychiatrist and a Pediatrician Look at Modern Baby and Child Care," LLLI Information Sheet #201-6/64, La Leche League International, Inc. p. 4.
59. Jimmy Lynn Avery, "Closet Nursing: A Symptom of Intolerance and a Forerunner of Social Change," *Keeping Abreast Journal* 2:3, 1977, p. 212.

60. *La Leche League Love Story,* op. cit., p. 23.
61. Viva, "Hooked on Weaning," excerpt from *The Baby, Ms,* April 1975, pp. 51–54.
62. Letters, *Ms,* August 1975, pp. 6–8.
63. Judith Lumley and Jill Astbury, *Birth Rites, Birth Rights* (West Melbourne, Thomas Nelson, Australia, 1980), p. 199.
64. Blachman, op. cit., p. 286.
65. Rothman, op. cit., p. 184.
66. Janet B. Younger, "The Management of Night Waking in Older Infants," *Pediatric Nursing,* May/June 1982, p. 157.
67. Elly Rakowitz and Gloria S. Rubin, *Living with Your New Baby* (New York, Watts, 1978), p. 180.
68. Report of the Eleventh Ross Roundtable on Critical Approaches to Common Pediatric Problems, *Counseling the Mother on Breast Feeding* (Columbus Ross Labs, Ohio 43216, 1980) p. 14.
69. Ibid., p. 14.
70. Joseph McFalls, "Where Have All the Children Gone?" *Human Sexuality* (Sluice Dock, Conn., Duskin Publications, 1981/82) p. 90.
71. Merilyn Solomon et al., "Breastfeeding, Natural Mothering, and Working Outside of the Home," *20th Century Obstetrics Now* Volume 2, op. cit., pp. 475–506.
72. Lynn Moen files, Seattle, Wash. 1965.
73. Interview with Margot Edwards, 1981.
74. Mary White, *Leaven,* Franklin Park, Ill., March/April 1976.
75. *La Leche League News,* op. cit., May/June 1976.
76. Quoted in David Stewart, *The Five Standards for Safe Childbearing* (P.O. Box 428, Marble Hill, Mo., NAPSAC Publications, 1981), p. i.
77. Pat Stone, "Marian Tompson," *Mother Earth News,* Sept/October 1982, p. 17.
78. Marian Tompson, letter to Margot Edwards, op. cit., p. 1.
79. Stone, op. cit., p. 17.
80. Elisabeth Bing, "The Future of Childbirth Education," *Self, Family, Society: Toward Freedom and Growth in Parenthood* (CEA of Seattle, 1976), p. 63, out of print.

## CHAPTER FOUR

1. Editorial, "New Science of Birth," *Newsweek,* November 15, 1976, reprinted in *Readings in Human Development 78/79* (Sluice Dock, Conn., Duskin, 1978), pp. 40, 42.
2. Alice Lake, "Childbirth in America," *McCall's,* January 1976, reprinted in *Readings in Early Childhood Education 77/78* (Sluice Dock, Conn., Duskin, 1977), pp. 62–65.
3. Logan Clendening, *The Romance of Medicine* (New York, Garden City Publishing Co., 1933), p. 145.
4. Edward Shorter, *A History of Women's Bodies* (New York, Basic Books, 1982), pp. 81–82; and Clendening, op. cit., p. 144.
5. Clendening, op. cit., pp. 146, 147, 149.
6. Anthony Smith, *The Body* (New York, Walker and Company, 1968), p. 143.
7. Clendening, op. cit., pp. 146–147.
8. Smith, op. cit., pp. 145–146.
9. Smith, op. cit., p. 145.
10. Harold Speert, *Obstetrics and Gynecology in America: A History* (One East

Wacker Drive, Chicago, American College of Obstetricians and Gynecologists, 1980), p. 38.

11. Ibid., p. 49.

12. Ibid., p. 54.

13. Ibid., p. 52.

14. Ibid., p. 51.

15. Llaminaria tents to dilate the cervix were also used by abortionists. See Shorter, op. cit., p. 149.

16. Speert, op. cit., pp. 46, 48; and Barbara Ehrenreich and Dierdre English, *Complaints and Disorders: The Sexual Politics of Sickness* (Old Westbury, New York, The Feminist Press, 1973), pp. 34–35.

17. Joseph B. DeLee, *Obstetrics for Nurses* (Philadelphia, W. B. Saunders, 1916), pp. 197, 193.

18. Speert, op. cit., pp. 184–185. The use of external version to turn the breech is making a comeback in the eighties because under certain conditions it is safer than a cesarean section. See note 58.

19. Grace Abbott and Frances Perkins, *Maternal Mortality in Fifteen States* (Washington, D.C., Children's Bureau, U.S. Department of Labor, 1933), p. 31. Courtesy of contributing author, Margaret Swigart, M.D., Pacific Grove, CA.

20. Quoted in Judy Litoff, *American Midwives: 1860 to the Present* (Westport, Conn., Greenwood Press, 1981), p. 67. See DeLee, *Obstetrics for Nurses*, op. cit., pp. 18–19: "The nurse may do much to aid the physician in obtaining from the public recognition for obstetrics that the specialty justly deserves. . . . The nurse may smooth the path for the advance of the obstetric art."

21. Iain Chalmers and Martin Richards, "Intervention and Causal Inference in Obstetric Practice," *Benefits and Hazards of the New Obstetrics* (Philadelphia, J. B. Lippincott, 1977), p. 40.

22. Robert E. Hall, *Nine Months' Reading* (Garden City, N.Y., Doubleday, 1973), pp. 103–104.

23. Of particular interest is Helen Wessel's *Under the Apple Tree: Marrying, Birthing, Parenting* (P.O. Box 9883, Fresno, CA 93795, Apple Tree Family Ministries, 1981). Wessel, a Christian feminist and past president of ICEA (1964–1966), studied the Greek language in order to counteract the belief that the pain of childbirth was divinely ordained.

24. Leabah H. Winter, *Consumer Guide to Health Care Costs*, (Sacramento, Cal., California Health Facilities Commission, 1982), p. 45.

25. Ibid., p. 45.

26. Suzanne Arms, letters, *Birth and the Family Journal*, Fall 1974, p. 13.

27. Michael Woods, "Resurgence Reported in Medical Malpractice Suits," *Monterey Peninsula Herald*, February 24, 1983.

28. See "Malpractice Suits Spark Costly Tests, Survey Says," *Monterey Peninsula Herald*, September 8, 1983, p. 7; and Margo Burke, "Woman Doctor-Lawyer Unafraid to Take on Medical Establishment," *Monterey Peninsula Herald*, November 6, 1983. Burke quoted Roberta Ritter, M.D., J.D., as saying she'd been so "appalled" by the 1973–4 malpractice crises that she founded a concensus group for medical accountability that led to work with the California Trial Lawyers' Association. The first woman to head the association, she said at a statewide meeting that she believed "only a small percentage of medical malpractice is recognized by patients . . . "

29. Leena Valvanne, interview with Mary Waldorf, Helsinki, Finland, 1981.

30. Sheryle Paukert, "One Hospital's Experience with the Implementation of Family Centered Maternity Care," *Journal of Obstetrical and Gynecological Nursing*, November/December 1979, pp. 351–358.

31. Roberto Caldeyro-Barcia, "Some Consequences of Obstetrical Interference"; "The Influence of Maternal Position on Time of Spontaneous Rupture of the Membranes, Progress of Labor, and Fetal Head Compression"; and "The Influence of Maternal Bearing Down Efforts during Second Stage on Fetal Well-being," *Birth* (110 El Camino Real, Berkeley, Cal. 94705), Reprints: $2.

32. Quoted in *Pregnant Women and Newborn Infants in California: A Deepening Crisis in Health Care* (Sacramento, Cal., California Department of Consumer Affairs, 1982), p. 134.

33. David Banta and Stephen Thacker, *Costs and Benefits of Electronic Fetal Monitoring: A Review of the Literature* (U.S. Department of HEW, Public Health Service, 3700 East West Highway, Hyattsville, Md. 20782, PHS 79-3245, 1979).

34. *National Institute of Child Health and Development Report on EFM* (Office of Research, NICHD, Bl. 31, Rm. 2A34, Bethesda, Md. 20014, 1979).

35. Speert, op. cit., pp. 222–223.

36. Elliot McLearey, *New Miracles of Childbirth* (New York, David Mckay, 1974), p. 10.

37. J. R. Murphy, "The Relationship of Electronic Fetal Monitoring Patterns to Infant Outcome Measures in a Random Sample of Term Size Infants Born to High Risk Mothers," *American Journal of Epidemiology*, October 1981, pp. 534–548. Murphy repeated trials pioneered by Albert Haverkamp that demonstrated EFM to have little predictive value in determining fetal outcome. See A. D. Haverkamp et al., "The Evaluation of Continuous Heart Rate Monitoring in High Risk Pregnancy," *American Journal of Obstetrics and Gynecology*, Volume 125, June 1, 1976, pp. 310–320; A. D. Haverkamp et al., "A Controlled Trial of Differential Effects of Intrapartum Monitoring," *American Journal of Obstetrics and Gynecology*, Volume 134, June 15, 1979, pp. 399–412. See also A. D. Haverkamp and M. Orleans, "An Assessment of Electronic Fetal Monitoring," *Obstetrical Intervention and Technology in the 80s*, edited by Diony Young (New York, Haworth Press, 1982). Since this data indicates that EFM cannot accurately predict brain damage but only the possibility of fetal distress, some experts believe another test, fetal blood sampling, should be used in conjunction with EFM to determine fetal blood pH or acidity. A pH of 7.2 or lower for two consecutive tests is a reliable indicator of acidosis, which occurs with anoxia, and signals the need for the baby to be born as quickly as possible, usually by cesarean. If the pH is normal, labor may continue, and the woman is spared unnecessary surgery. Unfortunately, because of expense, many community hospitals without doctors on call to perform this simple, rapid test, do not maintain labs and staff for fetal blood sampling.

38. P. Budetti et al., "The Cost Effectiveness of Neonatal Intensive Care," Health Policy Program, University of California, San Francisco. Performed under contract #433-22-60.0 for the Office of Technology Assessment, U.S. Congress, February 22, 1980, p. 45.

39. David Banta, "Electronic Fetal Monitoring: Is It of Benefit?" *Birth and the Family Journal*, Winter 1979, p. 240.

40. Howard Brody and James R. Thompson, "The Maximin Strategy in Modern Obstetrics," *Journal of Family Practice*, Volume 12 (16), 1981.

41. Kathleen Newland, "Infant Mortality and the Health of Societies," *World Watch Report* 47 (1776 Massachusetts Ave N.W., Washington, D.C. 20036, Worldwatch Institute, 1982).

42. M. Hack et al., "Changing Trends of Neonatal and Postneonatal Deaths in Very Low Birth Weight Infants," *American Journal of Obstetrics and Gynecology*, August 1980, pp. 797–800. See David Stewart, *The Five Standards for Safe*

*Childbearing* (P.O. Box 428, Marble Hill, Mo. 63764, NAPSAC Publications, 1981), pp. 430–452, and Iain Chalmers, "The Search for Indices," *The Lancet*, November 17, 1979, pp. 1063 and 1064, who assert that statistics on infant mortality are misleading when deaths at different ages are lumped together. For example, "infant mortality," refers to deaths following live births in the first year of life, and includes deaths caused by birth problems, infectious diseases, sudden infant deaths, and deaths resulting from poverty, abuse and/or neglect. Another category, "perinatal death," refers to deaths occurring in the first twenty-eight days of life, including stillbirths, fetal mortalities (death of fetus older than twenty weeks gestation), and neonatal mortalities (death of child weighing over five hundred grams within twenty-eight days). In making comparisons, these categories are sometimes mistakenly used interchangeably.

43. Not only are categories of statistics sometimes misused, but scientists do not always agree on which method of research gives the best results. See Iain Chalmers, "Scientific Inquiry and Authoritarianism in Perinatal Care and Education," *Birth*, Fall 1983, pp. 151–164, in which Chalmers claims that randomized controlled trials are the most scientific and unbiased form of research because of their random element. Others think it unethical to subject humans to drugs or interventions that, on one hand, might deprive them of a potentially helpful drug or device or, on the other, might cause harm if administered. Scientists who favor the trials, like long-time ASPO and ICEA supporter Dr. Murray Enkin, respond that without the trials, technology will be used without adequate prior testing, as in the case of EFM. (Interview with Margot Edwards, 1981).

44. Judith Lumley, "The Irresistible Rise of Electronic Fetal Monitoring," *Birth: Issues in Perinatal Care and Education*, Fall 1982, pp. 150–151.

45. Yvonne Brackbill, "Effects of Obstetric Medication on Fetus and Infant, "*Handbook of Infant Development*, edited by J. D. Osofsky (New York, Wiley, 1978).

46. "Pain Killers in Labor: 'Caution Flag is Up'," *Medical World News*, February 5, 1979, pp. 23–24.

47. Quoted in Richard Hughes, "Brain Damage in Babies Tied to Anesthesia," *Washington Star Ledger*, January 14, 1979, p. 53.

48. Doris Haire, "How the FDA Determines the Safety of Drugs: Just How Safe is Safe?" National Women's Health Network, 224 7th St. SE, Washington, D.C. 20003. $1.

49. Quoted in Ann Gray, "FDA Withholds Drug Risks from Public," *The Federal Monitor*, Alexandria, Va., August 30, 1981, p. 1.

50. Helen Marieskind, *An Evaluation of Cesarean Section in the United States*, U.S. Department of HEW, Washington, D.C. 1979, and Michael Woods, "Americans Increasingly Captivated by Surgery," *Monterey Peninsula Herald*, May 2, 1982.

51. Gena Corea, "The Cesarean Epidemic," *Mother Jones*, July 1980, p. 31.

52. Speert, op. cit., p. 150.

53. Judith Lumley, *Birth Rites, Birth Rights* (West Melbourne, Thomas Nelson, Australia, 1980), p. 123.

54. Murray Enkin, "Having a Section is Having a Baby," *Birth and the Family Journal*, Fall 1977, pp. 103, 105. See William H. Spellacy, *OB/Gyn News*, Volume 16 (22), November 1981, who found that up to one-third of a group of prematures in an intensive care nursery were there because of ill-timed cesareans.

55. Deanne Bunce, "Cesarean Section: The Latest Trend in Childbirth Alternatives," *Second Opinion*, Coalition for the Medical Rights of Women, Fall 1979.

56. Helen Marieskind, *Women in the Health Care System: Patients, Providers, and Programs* (St. Louis, C. V. Mosby, 1980), p. 255.

57. Ibid., pp. 255–256.

58. See Kirk A. Keegan, Jr., "Changing Trends in Cesarean Section," *Western Symposium on Maternal-Child Health*, (Anaheim, Cal., March 7, 1981), pp. 46–52, for recommendations made by the Task Force on Cesarean Birth about vaginal delivery of the breech. Breeches accounted for 15.7 percent of the total increase in cesarean, and this rise was rationalized on the basis of findings in older research that showed vaginal breech delivery to be highly dangerous. However, as Keegan explained, the Task Force said surgery should be done more selectively because the research was flawed, magnifying the risk rate. Earlier research did not differentiate between premature and full-term infant outcome, nor between different types of breech presentation. Keegan presented Task Force criteria for safe vaginal delivery of the frank breech: fetal head well-flexed, weight under eight pounds, normal maternal pelvis, good progress in labor, and a skilled physician. Dr. Harlan A. Ellis of Visalia, CA, who has delivered hundreds of breech babies safely, maintains a similar eligibility criteria (although he accepts as safe, infants weighing between five and a half and eight and a half pounds). He does require that parents requesting vaginal delivery of the breech be educated in childbirth beforehand. Since all his patients receive childbirth education as part of the prenatal care package, mothers with unexpected breech presentations are not disqualified for vaginal delivery on that basis only. (Interview with Margot Edwards, 1983.)

59. Elizabeth Connor Shearer, "A Special Interest Group Brings About Change," *Birth Control and Controlling Birth*, edited by Helen C. Holmes et al., (Clifton, N.J., The Humana Press, 1980), p. 281.

60. Elizabeth Connor Shearer, "NIH Concensus Development Task Force on Cesarean Childbirth: The Process and the Result," *Birth and the Family Journal*, Spring 1981, p. 30.

61. Nancy Wainer Cohen and Lois J. Estner, *Silent Knife: Cesarean Prevention and Vaginal Birth After Cesarean* (Massachusetts, Bergen and Garvey, 1983), p. 3.

62. Marieskind, op. cit., p. 255.

63. Quoted in Margaret Hickey, "Training for Childbirth," *Ladies' Home Journal*, May 1953, p. 146.

64. Marieskind, op. cit., p. 255.

65. Joan Arehard-Treichel, "Fetal Ultrasound: How Safe?", *Science News*, June 12, 1982, pp. 396–397.

66. Max Baker et al., "Safe or Sorry: Exposure to Radiation," *Pediatric Nursing*, July/August 1982, pp. 237–243.

67. Mel Stratmeyer, "Research in Ultrasound Bioeffects: A Public Health View," *Birth and the Family Journal*, Summer 1980, pp. 92–100.

68. *Carcinogen Information Bulletin*, (Washington University, St. Louis, Mo., 63130, Center for the Biology of Natural Systems, July 1980), p. 1.

69. William O'Brien, *OB/Gyn News*, July 15, 1979, p. 3.

70. Arehard-Treichel, op. cit., p. 398.

71. "Ultrasound Exams Reveal Sex of Fetus," *Monterey Peninsula Herald*, October 25, 1983, p. 8.

72. Barbara Bolson, "Question of Risk Still Hovers Over Routine Prenatal Risk of Ultrasound," *Journal of American Medical Association*, April 23/30, 1982, p. 2195.

73. Quoted in *Pregnant Women*, op. cit., p. 144.

74. Gail and Tom Brewer, *The Brewer Medical Diet for Normal and High-Risk Pregnancy* (New York, Simon and Schuster, 1983).

75. Phillip Rhodes "Human Relations in Obstetrics," quoted in *AIMS Quarterly Journal*, 67 Lennox Road, London, Spring 1982, p. 1.
76. Catherine Boyd and Lea Sellers, *The British Way of Birth* (London, Pan Books Ltd., 1981), p. 112.
77. Valerie Grove, "Mother-to-Be Knows Best," *London Evening Standard*, March 18, 1982, p. 24.
78. Quoted in Grove, ibid., p. 24.
79. "Birth Rights Rally," *New Generation*, (London, National Childbirth Trust, June 1982), p. 6, 7.
80. Ibid., p. 7.
81. Quoted in Debora Moggach, *London Times*, November 9, 1980, p. 108.
82. Ibid.
83. Sheila Kitzinger, *The Experience of Childbirth* (New York, Penguin 1978), p. 24.
84. Adrienne Rich, "Theft of Childbirth," *Seizing Our Bodies*, edited by Claudia Dreifus (New York, Vintage, 1977), p. 152.
85. Sheila Kitzinger, *Women As Mothers* (New York, Random House, 1978), p. 122.
86. Iain Chalmers, "Implications of the Current Debate on Obstetric Practice," *The Place of Birth*, edited by Sheila Kitzinger and John A. Davis (Oxford, Oxford University Press, 1978), pp. 44–54.
87. Harry Oxorn, *Human Labor and Birth* (New York, Appleton-Century Crofts, 1980), pp. 460–461.
88. Doris Haire, *The Cultural Warping of Childbirth* (P.O. Box 40048, Minneapolis, Minn. 55420, ICEA Publications, 1972), p. 24.
89. Shelly Romalis, "Natural Childbirth and the Reluctant Physician," *Childbirth: Alternatives to Medical Control*, edited by Shelly Romalis (Austin, University of Texas Press, 1981), p. 76.
90. Michelle Harrison, *A Woman in Residence* (New York, Random House, 1982), p. 177.
91. David Banta and Stephen Thacker, "The Risks and Benefits of Episiotomy," *Birth: Issues in Perinatal Care and Education*, Spring 1982, pp. 25–30.
92. Rosemary Cogan, "The Unkindest Cut," *Contemporary Obstetrics and Gynecology*, Volume 9, 1977, pp. 55–59. See David Privor quoted in *Childbirth Without Pain Education Association News*, (Detroit, November 1981, p. 1) who said that he transferred from a system of care that always used routine episiotomies to one that largely avoids them. Dr. Privor, a friend to CEA San Diego, prefers the side-lying position for delivery and has observed, but not proven, that slowing of the fetal heart tones often occurs in second stage without damage to the baby.
93. *Maternal Health and Childbirth* (224 Seventh Street, Washington, D.C. 20003, National Women's Health Network, 1980), p. 1.

# CHAPTER FIVE

1. Quoted in *Birth Control and Controlling Birth*, edited by Helen B. Holmes et al. (Clifton, N.J., The Humana Press, 1980), p. 264.
2. A contemporary attack is contained in Edward Shorter's *The History of Women's Bodies* (New York, Basic Books, 1982). Shorter's picture of the old-time midwife reinforces conventional medical history. She was not only dirty and ignorant, but because of her unschooled haste, a dangerous interventionist.

This argument is a direct refutation of the work of feminist scholars and historians Gena Corea, Barbara Ehrenreich, Dierdre English, Adrienne Rich, Dorothy Wertz, and others. Shorter's case, built on reports made mainly by doctors in French and German communities in the seventeenth and eighteenth centuries, is open to the charge that the medical writers may have been biased in their view of the competition. Professional historians have questioned his methods and conclusions on other grounds as well. See letters, *Birth*, Spring 1984.

3. Barbara Ehrenreich and Dierdre English, *Witches, Midwives, and Nurses* (Old Westbury, N.Y., The Feminist Press, 1973), p. 7. While most historians agree that a great fear and hatred of women marked the European witch craze, few accept the argument that persecution was designed by church and nobility to destroy peasant organizations, especially the community of women healers. Traditional theories have ranged from Hugh Trevor-Roper's explanation of the craze as fall out from religious wars, to Keith Thomas' belief that the rise of capitalism produced mass guilt over economic inequity, prompting the need for scapegoats. One of the most interesting theories was offered in 1982 by Stanislav Andreski who connected persecution with the sudden appearance of syphilis in late fifteenth-century Europe. This would partially explain the focus on women witches (85 percent of the trial victims are estimated to have been female) since in a patriarchal society, women were assumed to be the source of the infection and its dreadful aftermath of dementia, paralysis, stillbirths and deformed offspring. Some feminist historians such as Andrea Dworkin follow Margaret Murray's lead earlier in the century in proposing that many women were actually holding sabbats and worshiping old gods in pagan cults that had survived the Christian era. According to this theory, the ability of the women to use herbs and drugs for hallucination as well as healing, and their knowledge of childbirth and abortion, made them an intolerable threat to the Church and its inquisitors. See Hugh R. Trevor-Roper, *The European Witchcraze of the Sixteenth and Seventeenth Centuries* (New York, Harper & Row, 1967); Keith Thomas, *Religion and the Decline of Magic* (London, Oxford University Press, 1972); Stanislav Andreski, "The Syphilitic Shock," *Encounter*, May 1982, pp. 7–25; Andrea Dworkin, *Woman Hating* (New York, Dutton, 1974).

4. Quoted in Fran Ventre, "Midwifery in America: A Brief History," *Family Journal*, May 1981, p. 20.

5. Anthony Smith, *The Body* (New York, Garden City Publications, 1968), p. 141.

6. Harold Speert *Obstetrics and Gynecology in America: a History*, (One East Wacker Drive, Chicago, American College of Obstetricians and Gynecologists, 1980), p. 6.

7. Ibid., p. 9.

8. Quoted in Speert, op. cit., p. 10. For details on the Hutchinson trial, see "The Examination of Mrs. Ann Hutchinson at the Court of Newton," *Root of Bitterness*, edited by Nancy F. Cott (New York, Dutton, 1972). pp. 34–36.

9. Quoted in Speert, op. cit., p. 11.

10. Quoted in Jean Donnison, *Midwives and Medical Men: A History of Inter-Professional Rivalries and Women's Rights* (New York, Schocken, 1977), p. 33.

11. Quoted in Speert, op. cit., p. 139.

12. Quoted in Barbara Ehrenreich and Dierdre English, *For Her Own Good* (Garden City, NY, Anchor/Doubleday, 1978), p. 42.

13. Ann Gray, "How Doctors Use Government to Maintain a Monopoly and What Consumers Can Do About It," *Compulsory Hospitalization or Freedom of*

*Choice in Childbirth*, Volume 1, edited by David and Lee Stewart, (P.O. Box 428, Marble Hill, MO 63764, NAPSAC Publications, 1979), pp. 13–22. Paul Starr, in *The Social Transformation of American Medicine* (New York, Basic Books, 1983), pp. 106–127, has another interpretation of the events related to medical licensing and regulation. According to his research, regulars "set aside their scruples about consorting with heretics and made common cause" with irregular homeopaths and eclectics to control entry into the profession. However, by 1900 irregulars lost their appeal in the wake of scientific medical advancement such as antiseptic surgery and X-ray.

14. Dorothy Wertz, "Man-Midwifery," *Birth Control and Controlling Birth*, op. cit., p. 153.

15. Barbara Ehrenreich and Deidre English, *Complaints and Disorders: The Politics of Sickness* (Old Westbury, New York, The Feminist Press, 1973), p. 42.

16. Quoted in "Perils of American Women," *Root of Bitterness*, edited by Nancy F. Cott (New York, Dutton, 1972), p. 296.

17. Catherine Beecher, "On Female Health in America," *Root of Bitterness*, op. cit., pp. 263–265.

18. Quoted in David Stewart, *NAPSAC News*, Fall 1981, p. 8.

19. Quoted in *For Her Own Good*, op. cit., p. 86.

20. Ibid.

21. Speert, op. cit., p. 15.

22. Ibid., p. 147.

23. Neil Devitt, "How Doctors Conspired to Eliminate the Midwife Even Though the Scientific Data Supports Midwifery," *Compulsory Hospitalization or Freedom of Choice in Childbirth*, Volume 2, op. cit., pp. 345–370.

24. Gay Courter, *The Midwife* (Boston, Houghton-Mifflin, 1981).

25. Devitt, op. cit., pp. 354–356.

26. Quoted in Speert, op. cit., p. 144. Although the Sheppard-Towner Bill passed in 1921, it was originally introduced in 1918 by Representative Jeanette Rankin of Montana, who along with feminist supporters became the target of the AMA. Although physicians bitterly opposed government support of nursing and public health programs designed in part to upgrade midwifery, the bill re-introduced in 1921 passed with support from activist women, the Children's Bureau, the Department of Agriculture, and the American Federation of Labor. However, by the end of the decade, doctors persuaded government that the funds should go for medical research, not to public health nurses and midwives, because childbirth belonged in the medical domain. See Phyllis Sawyer Williams, ICEA *Sharing*, January 1981, p. 2.

27. Kathy Kahn, *Hillbilly Women* (New York, Avon, 1972), p. xiv.

28. David Stewart, *The Five Standards of Safe Childbearing* (P.O. Box 428, Marble Hill Mo. 63764, NAPSAC Publications, 1981), p. 21.

29. Barbara Brennan and Joan Rattner Hellman, *The Complete Book of Midwifery* (New York, Dutton, 1973), p. 12.

30. Raven Lang, *Birth Book* (Ben Lomond, Cal., Genesis, 1972), unpaged.

31. Marshall Klaus and John Kennell, *Parent Infant Bonding* (New York, Mosby, 1982). The Klaus-Kennell work originally appeared as "Maternal Attachment: Importance of First Postpartum Days," *New England Journal of Medicine*, Volume 286, March 2, 1972. However, a nurse, Reva Rubin, preceded Klaus with the bonding theory in 1963. See Reva Rubin, "Maternal Touch," *Nursing Outlook*, Volume 11 (11), 1963, pp. 828–831.

32. The risks of induction and augmentation of labor with a pitocin drip include increased maternal pain, higher usage of analgesia and anesthesia, and three times as many neonatal respiratory problems. See M. P. M. Richards, "A Place of Safety? An Exam of the Risks of Hospital Delivery," *Place of Birth*,

edited by Sheila Kitzinger and John A. Davis (London, Oxford University Press, 1978), p. 76; and Constance Bean, *Labor and Delivery: An Observer's Diary* (New York, Doubleday, 1977), pp. 130–137. To assist others who want to found freestanding birth centers, the Maternity Center established the National Association of Childbearing Centers, R.D.1, Box 1, Perkiomenville, Pa. 18074. (215) 234-8068. An informational packet costs $15.

33. Louis E. Mehl, "Complications of Home Birth: an Analysis of 287 Consecutive Home Births from Santa Cruz County, California," *Birth and the Family Journal*, Summer, 1975, pp. 123–135. See follow-up studies: Mehl et al., "Outcomes of Elective Home Births: A Series of 1146 Cases," *Journal of Reproductive Medicine*, Volume 19, 1977, pp. 281–290; and Mehl, "Evaluations of Outcomes of Non-Nurse Midwives: Matched Comparisons with Physicians," *Women and Health*, Summer 1980.

34. Raven Lang, op. cit.

35. Ibid.

36. Raven Lang, interview with Margot Edwards and Mary Waldorf, 1979.

37. "More Specific Charges Asked Against Midwives," *Santa Cruz Sentinel*, June 16, 1974.

38. "Midwife Suspects to Appear," *Santa Cruz Sentinel*, August 2, 1974.

39. "Court Rules for the Midwives," *Santa Cruz Sentinel*, February 6, 1976, p. 1.

40. "DA Drops Midwife Case," *Santa Cruz Sentinel*, December 9, 1976.

41. "Case of the Midwife Charged with Murder," *San Jose Mercury News*, December 3, 1978, p. 7L.

42. Ibid.

43. Mark Hunter, "Mothers and Outlaws," *New West*, December 22, 1980, p. 68.

44. Ibid., p. 62.

45. David Peterson, letter to Tarpening Supporters, 1979.

46. Mark Hunter, op. cit., p. 68.

47. Ibid., p. 75.

48. Ibid.

49. The California Association for Midwives (CAM) (P.O. Box 3306, San Jose, Cal. 95156), assembled a list of California midwives in trouble with the law from 1974 to 1983, available by request for mailing costs.

50. ACHI Press Release, International Headquarters, P.O. Box 39498, Los Angeles, Cal. 90039, 1981.

51. Quoted in David Stewart, "The Conspiracy of Doctors Against Midwives," *NAPSAC News*, Fall 1981, p. 8.

52. *NAACOG Bulletin*, June 1981.

53. Suzanne Arms, *Immaculate Deception* (Boston, Houghton-Mifflin, 1975), p. 54.

54. Angela Davis in *Pregnant Women and Newborn Infants in California: A Deepening Crises in Health Care* (Sacramento, Cal., California State Department of Consumer Affairs, March 26, 1982), p. 26.

55. *Pregnant Women*, op. cit., p. ii.

56. Ibid., p. 219.

57. David Osborne, "My Wife, the Doctor," *San Francisco Chronicle-Examiner*, April 3, 1983, p. 9.

58. *Pregnant Women*, op. cit., p. xx.

59. Ibid., p. 135.

60. Ibid., p. 136.

61. Ibid., p. 143.

62. Ibid., pp. 301, xi.

63. Ibid., p. xi.

64. Diane Divoky, "Perinatal Care Bypasses the Poor," *The Sacramento Bee*, February 2, 1981, p. B-2.

65. *Pregnant Women*, op. cit., p. 182.
66. Michael Krisman, Deputy Director of California DCA, 1020 N St. Sacramento CA 95814, letter to midwife supporters, May 29, 1980.
67. Quoted in *Pregnant Women*, op. cit., pp. 165–166.
68. B. S. Levy, "Reducing Neonatal Mortality Rates with Nurse Midwives," *American Journal of Obstetrics and Gynecology*, January 1971, pp. 50–58.
69. *Pregnant Women*, op. cit., p. 184.
70. Patricia McCarty, "Nurse Midwives Forced Out of Practice," *The American Nurse*, Kansas City, Spring 1981, p. 12.
71. *Trade Regulation Reports #559*, Commerce Clearing House, Inc., Publisher of Topical Law Reports, 4025 W. Peterson Avenue, Chicago, IL 60646, September 13, 1982.
72. Bill Snyder, "Senate Antitrust Vote Called Total Defeat for Doctors' Group," *Nashville Banner*, December 21, 1982, p. 6-C. Another victory for the nurse midwives occured when a physician-owned insurance company was warned again that it could not drop insurance coverage on doctors who provide backup for nursemidwives. See Carolyn Shoulders, "Insure MDs Who Oversee Midwives, Firm Repeatedly Told," *Tennessean*, April 20, 1983, pp. 1, 4.
73. Harriet Palmer and Liz Summerhayes, interviews with Margot Edwards, San Jose, CA, April 1983.
74. Discussion (anonymous speaker) at Technological Approaches to Obstetrics: Benefits, Risks, Alternatives III, San Francisco, March 18, 1983.
75. Editorial, *ACOG News*, reprinted in NAPSAC News, Spring 1982, p. 5. The attitude expressed in the ACOG editorial was attacked by Robert M. Cunningham, editor of *Modern Hospital* in 1967: "Lay interference is a fundamental principle of American life. It . . . puts civilians in charge of our military . . . makes teachers and education administrators responsive to the demands of boards of education . . . gives the electorate the final authority over all public officials. . . . A doctor who objects to lay interference as such is asking that the medical profession be given the status of an untouchable priesthood." Quoted by Fred Cook, *The Plot Against the Patient* (Clifton, N.J., Prentice-Hall, 1967), p. 281.
76. Dan J. Tannenhouse, "Liability and the Omission of Obstetric Procedures Thought to be of No Benefit," Presentation at Technological Approaches, op. cit.
77. John Grad, "Hospitals and Obstetric Specialty Restraints on Primary Practitioners: Avenues for Redress," Presentation at Technological Approaches, op. cit.
78. Charles Petit, "Midwives' Good Record at San Francisco General," *San Francisco Chronicle*, August 7, 1981, p. 22.
79. Raymond Devries, "The Alternative Birth Center: Option or Cooption?" *Women and Health* 5:3, 1980, pp. 47–60.
80. Gary Richwald, "Home Vs. Hospital," *Compulsory Hospitalization*, Volume 2, op. cit., p. 470.
81. Ruth Lubic Watson, "Alternatives in Maternity Care," *Childbirth: Alternatives to Medical Control* (Austin, University of Texas Press, 1981), p. 227.
82. Ibid., p. 241. See also Childbirth Alternatives Quarterly Spring 1983, pp. 4–9 for history and experiences of induced labor. (CAQ, Bin 62 S.L.A.C., Stanford, Cal.)
83. Ina May Gaskin, "Community Alternatives in High Technology Birth," *Birth Control and Controlling Birth*, op. cit., p. 227.
84. Billye Y. Avery and Judith M. Levy, "Hospital and Birth Center Contrasts," *Birth Control and Controlling Birth*, op. cit., p. 235.
85. Ruth Wilf, "Fulfilling the Needs of Families in a Hospital Setting: Can It Be Done?" *20th Century Obstetrics Now*, Volume 1, edited by David and Lee

Stewart (P.O. Box 428, Marble Hill, Mo. 63764, NAPSAC Publications, 1977) p. 47.

86. Ruth Wilf, interview with Mary Waldorf and Margot Edwards, Monterey, CA, May 1983.

87. Rajima Baldwin, *Special Delivery* (231 Adrian Rd., Milbrae, Cal. 94030, Le Femme Press, 1979).

# CONCLUSION

1. Quoted in Catherine R. Stimpson, "Gerda Lerner on the Future of Our Past," *Ms*, September 1981, p. 95.

2. Norma Swenson, "Childbirth Overview," *Birth Control and Controlling Birth*, edited by Helen B. Holmes et al. (Clifton, N.J., The Humana Press, 1980), p. 145.

3. Quoted in Barbara Ehrenreich and Deidre English, *For Her Own Good* (Garden City, N.Y., Doubleday, 1978), p. 97.

4. Michelle Harrison, *A Woman in Residence* (New York, Random House, 1982), p. 125.

5. Diana Scully, *Men Who Control Women's Health* (Boston, Houghton Mifflin 1980), p. 15. Sources vary on the approximate number of women in medicine; the average is about twenty-five percent in the first year of medical school and fifteen to eighteen percent, depending on the specialty, in the graduating class.

6. Margaret Gamper, letter to Margot Edwards, July 1983.

7. Norma Swenson, "Procreation Politics," *Maternal Child Health and Childbirth*, *Resource Guide #4* (Washington, D.C., National Women's Health Network, 1980), p. 7, out of print.

8. See Nancy Stoller Shaw, *Forced Labor: Maternity Care in the United States* (Elmsford, N.Y., Pergamon, 1974); Diana Scully, op. cit; Ann Oakley, *Women Confined* (New York, Shocken, 1980); and Barbara Katz Rothman, *In Labor: Women and Power in the Birthplace* (New York, W. W. Norton, 1982). Dr. Shaw and Dr. Oakley independently observed how hospitalized women were treated as subordinates by male doctors. Dr. Scully documented evidence that women's treatment preferences were secondary to student doctors' need for surgical experience. Dr. Rothman contrasted beliefs held by doctors and midwives about maternity care to show how beliefs influenced clinical practice.

9. Adrienne Rich, *Of Woman Born* (New York, Bantam Edition, 1977), p. 117.

10. Swenson, op. cit., p. 145.

11. Timothy D. Shelhardt, "Corporate PAC's Turning Attention to States as Deregulation Gains," *The Wall Street Journal*, October 28, 1982, p. 33.

12. Perry Garfinkel, "The Coming Battle Over Health Care," *Focus*, Publication of KQED, San Francisco, March 1983, p. 31.

13. Quoted in John Carlova, "Will Low-Cost Healers Replace M.D.s?" *Medical Economics*, August 9, 1982, p. 87.

14. Barry Vincour, "Reining in Health Care Costs," *Focus*, June 1980, p. 20.

15. Letters, "The Outpatient Solution to Rising Health Care Costs," *The New York Times*, April 13, 1983, p. 20.

16. Rose Kushner, *Why Me?, What Every Woman Should Know About Breast Cancer to Save her Life* (New York, New American Library, 1977).

17. Boston Women's Health Book Collective, *Our Bodies, Our Selves* (New York, Simon and Schuster, 1979), p. 13.

18. Gay Courter, letter to Margot Edwards, July 1983.
19. Genna Withrow, "Nurse and Non-Nurse Midwives Unite," *NAPSAC News*, Winter 1981, p. 1.
20. Ina May Gaskin, "MANA Update," *The Practicing Midwife*, Volume 1, No. 18, p. 2.
21. Elizabeth Davis, A Guide to Midwifery: Heart and Hands (P.O. Box 613, Santa Fe, N.M. 87501, John Muir Publication, 1981), p. 2.
22. Ehrenreich and English, op. cit., p. 292.

# INDEX

Accouchement force, 105
Addams, Jane 70-71
Aiken, Charlotte, 84, 85, 87
Alternative Birth Centers (ABCs), 182-3
Alternative Birth Crisis Coalition
(ABCC), 98
Alternative practitioners. *See* practitioners, mid-level and alternative
American Civil Liberties Union, 173
American College of Nurse-Midwives,
180, 194
American College of Obstetricians and
Gynecologists (ACOG), 10, 78, 177,
178, 181.
American Foundation for Maternal and
Child Health, 115; conference sponsorship, 117, 123
American Gynecological Society, 19th
century, 103-104
American Journal of Obstetrics and
Gynecology, 182-183
American Medical Association (AMA),
1, 4, 86; history, 151; opposition to
midwives and other practitioners 153,
154, 173, 178, 180, 193
American Society for Psychoprophylaxis
in Obstetrics (ASPO): origin, 48-50,
51-52. *See also* Lamaze method
Andreski, Stanislav, 208n.3
Anesthesia in childbirth. *See* drugs in
labor and delivery
Angoff, Jay, 180
Anoxia, 119. *See also* fetal distress
Arehart-Treichel, Joan, 130
Arms, Suzanne, 108, 174, 192
Association for Childbirth Education
(ACE), 61
Association for Childbirth at Home
(ACHI), 173
Avery, Billye Y., 185
Avery, Jimmy Lynn, 92

Baker, Josephine, 71, 154
Baldwin, Rajima, 188
Banta, David: review of EFM research,
5, 117-121
Barnes, Allan C., 54
Barrad, Gerold, 51
Baya, Carolle, 172
Beecher, Catherine, 152
Beischer, Norman, 124
Belski, Adam, 14
Benjamin, Lois, 40
Bennett, Linda, 164, 174
Berg, Alan, 89
Bing, Elisabeth, viii, 65, 189, 190; and

founding of ASPO, 47-52; life and
work, 33-40; publications, 51;
remarks on safety, 99
*Birth Atlas*, 14
*Birth Book* (Lang), 158, 163-164
Birth centers, free-standing: Booth,
185-186; Birthplace 185; Childbearing
Center, 13-14, 183-184; The Farm,
184-185; informational packet,
210n.82. *See also* Chicago Maternity
Center, and Santa Cruz Birth Center
Birth centers, in-hospital. *See* alternative
birth centers (ABCs)
*Birth: Issues in Perinatal Care and Education*,
109, 178, 181
Birth Home, 181
Birtheeze, 25
Blachman, Linda, 77, 93-94
Blackwell, Angela Glover, 75
Blessing Way, 187-188
Bolsen, Barbara, 131
Bonding theories, 94, 140, 159, 209n.31
Bonstein, Isadore, 47
Booth Maternity Hospital, 101, 185-186
Bottlefeeding: history, 69-72
Bowland, Kate, 164, 174
Boyd, Catherine, 132
Brackbill, Yvonne: research on long-term effects of obstetric drugs, 117,
121-123
Bradley Method, 33
Bradley, Robert, 27, 32-33, 85
Breastfeeding: decline among Black
women, 75; decline among middle-class women, 77-78; let-down reflex,
79-80; and maternal guilt, 93-95; sexual aspects, 90-91; in the Third
World, 72-75; weaning the older infant, 92-93; and working mothers,
95-97. *See also* infant formula controversy, and La Leche League International
Breech presentation: as indication for
cesarean section, 126, 206n.58 *See also*
version
Breckenridge, Mary, and FNS, 10-12
Brewer, Tom, 63
Brody, Howard, 120
Broman, Sarah H., 121
Bunce, Deanne, 125
Bureau of Medical Quality Assurance
(California) 164, 169, 192-193
Buxton, C. Lee 41-42, 55

California Medical Association, 177-178
Cesarean section: criteria, 206n.58; cur-

rent studies, 123-127; risk of prematurity, 205n.54; support groups, 125-126
Chabon, Irwin, 106
Chalmers, Iain, 141, 205n.42
Chamberlen, Peter, 101-102
Change in management of childbirth. *See* reform movement
Chicago Lying-in, 6, 9, 115
Chicago Maternity Center, 4, 6-10
Child abuse: "baby bopper detectives," 140
*Child Family Digest,* 84, 87
Childbearing Center, 183-184
Childbed fever. *See* puerperal fever
Childbirth. *See* consumers' rights in birth; control of birth; reform movement in childbirth; risks in childbirth; sexual aspects of childbirth
*Childbirth without Fear,* 14, 23, 36
The Childbirth Without Pain Education Association, 63
Children's Bureau, 4, 12, 105
"Closet Nursers," 92
Cobbett, William, 150
Cohen, Mme., vii, 43, 46, 49, 52
Cohen, Nancy Wainer, 125, 126
Coleman, Libby, 51
*Commonsense Childbirth* (Hazell), 65-66
Consumers' rights in birth, 106-107, 122-123. *See also* Department of Consumer Affairs hearings; Lester Hazell: life and work
Control of birth, 181; by hospital routine, 52-53; by obstetrician, 30, 138-140
Corbin, Hazel, 13, 48, 85
Corea, Gena, 3, 124
Costs of health care: as favoring reform, 193; as related to technology, 175-177
Counterstream research: definition, 116-117; report on research in four obstetrical technologies: EFM, obstetrical drugs, cesarean section, ultrasound, 117-132
Court cases. *See* midwife arrests in California; Nashville story. *See also* litigation
Courter, Gay, 154, 194
Cradleland. *See* Midwest Parentcraft Center
Cragin's Dictum, 127
Creevy, Don, 162
"Cruelty on the Maternity Wards" (Schultz) x, 55-57

C/SEC, 125-126
*The Cultural Warping of Childbirth,* (Haire) 109-110, 114
Cumings, Anne Flower: midwife defense, 165-166, 167, 170-171
Cunningham, Allan, 74

"Dancing in the Dark," (Blachman) 93-94
Daniels, Shari, 188
Davis, Angela, 175
Davis, Elizabeth, 195
Davis, Hope Valera, 173
Davis, John A., 141
Death Rates. *See* maternal mortality; infant mortality
De Kruif, Paul, 6-9, 17
DeLee, Joseph, B.: life and work, 4-6; theories and influence; 2, 9, 17, 24, 105
*The Delineator,* 71
Demmin, Tish, 173
Department of Consumer Affairs (California DCA), 164, hearings, 174-179
Department of Health, Education and Welfare, 117, 123
Devitt, Neil, 154
DeVries, Raymond, 183
Dickinson, Robert L., 14
Divorce: regarded by members of childbirth reform movement, 68
Donnison, Jean, 149-150
Doptone, 130. *See also* EFM
Doshi, Marianne, 167-168
Drugs in labor and delivery: controversy over use, 1930s, 1-3; history, 16-17, 150; long-term effects, 32-33, 52, 121-123; use in 20th century births, 11, 17-18, 31
Dworkin, Andrea, 208n.3
Dystocia: indication for cesarean section, 126

Edwards, Margot 97
Ehrenreich, Barbara, 76, 146, 195
Electronic fetal monitoring (EFM): description and scientific evaluation, 117-121; accuracy in indicating fetal distress, 119, 204n.37; related to improvement in infant mortality statistics,    119-121
Ellis, Harlan, 106, 206n.58
Empirics. *See* midwives
English, Dierdre, 76, 146,.195
Enkin, Murray, 106, 124, 205n.43

Episiotomy, 5; to avoid, 27, 207n.92; Kitzinger's experience with, 134; Lang's experience with, 159; politics of, 142-144; women's willingness to accept, 86

Ernst, Eunice, 11, 186

Erofeeva, N., 43

Estner, Lois J., 126

*Exercises for a True Natural Childbirth* (Hartman), 32

*Experience of Childbirth* (Kitzinger), 135, 141

Fairley, Jini, 125

Family-centered care, 62, 114-115, 189. *See also* alternative birth centers; AEC; ICEA

The Farm, 184-185

Farr, Minnie Mae, 155

Fathers in the delivery room, 26, 52. *See also* family-centered care

Federal Trade Commission anti-trust provisions, 180

Feminism: battle for freedom from labor pain 2-3; birth reform as a feminist concern, 63, 90, 97, 193-194; bottle-feeding as a symbol of freedom 77-78; women's liberation movements and reform, 97, 106, 144; recovery of women's history, vi, x-xi; 195. *See also* women

Fetal distress, 204n.37 *See also* risks in childbirth, infant

Fielding, Waldo, 40-41

Fistulas, 102, 104

Fitzhugh, Mabel, 85

Flexner report, 153

Food and Drug Administration (FDA): standards of safety, 122-123; study of ultrasound, 130; withdrawal of approval for elective oxytocin, 190

Forceps: American employment 19th and 20th centuries 103-106; component of prophylactic surgery, 5, 119; invention and early use, 101-102;

Franklin, John, 101, 185

Fraties, Gail Roy, 171

Friedan, Betty, 29

Froelich, Edwina, 88, 89

Frontier Nursing Service (FNS): history, 10-12. *See also* nurse-midwives

Fry, Fred, 64

Gamp, Sairy, 147-148

Gamper, Margaret, viii, 190; life and work, 18-28; membership in ICEA,

25, 63; publications, 25

Gamper Method, 24-28

Gaskin, Ina Mae, 184-185, 187

Gilliat, William, 16

*The Good Birth Guide* (Kitzinger), 141

Goodrich, Frederick, 48

Grace-New Haven Hospital, 31, 33

Graham, Sylvester, 151

Grove, Valerie, 132-133

Guttmacher, Alan, 37-38, 49

Gynecological surgery, 19th century, 104-105. *See also* hysterectomy

Gyorky, Paul, 89

Haire, Doris, viii-ix, 98, 144, 174, 189; *Cultural Warping of Childbirth*, 109-110, 114; life and work, 109-117; membership FDA consumer advisory committee, 122-123; research, 141, 142; support for counterstream research, 116-117; women's health, 144

Haire, John: co-author Doris Haire, 114; co-founder American Foundation, 115

Hamilton, Wallace B., 71-72, 76

*Harper's Bazaar*, 42, 47

Harrison, Michelle, 86-87, 143, 190

Hartman, Rhondda, 32, 65, 85

Haverkamp, Albert, 121, 204n.37

*Having a Baby after Thirty* (Bing and Coleman), 51

Hazell, Lester, ix, 97, 174, 191, 193; *Commonsense Childbirth*, 65-66; life and work, 57-68; midwife teacher, 68; observation of drugged birth, 31; teaching methods and philosophy, 64-66

Hazell, William: co-chairperson, ICEA, 15

Health industry, 191. *See also* medical-industrial alliance

Heardman, Helen, vii, 31-32, 85

Henderson, Victoria, 179-180

Heroic Medicine, 150

Hess, Amanda, 173

*The Hidden Malpractice*, (Corea) 124

*Hillbilly Women*, (Kahn) 155

Holmes, Oliver Wendell, 8

Holmes, Rudolph, 2

Holt, L. Emmett, 76, 94

Home birth: advocated by Lang and Santa Cruz midwives, 162-63; as regarded by La Leche League, 97; and NAPSAC, 97-98; statistics on safety, 9, 162, 185. *See also* ACHI; Chicago Maternity Center; FNS

Home birth, personal experience:

Hazell, 64; Kitzinger, 134; Lang, 186-187
Hommel, Flora, 63
Hunter, Mark, 171, 172
Hunter, William, 102
Husband-coached Childbirth (Bradley method), 33
"The Husband's Stitch," 143. *See also* episiotomy; sexual aspects of childbirth
Hutchinson, Anne, 148-149, 208n.8
Hysterectomy: Newton's studies, 86. *See also* gynecological surgery.

Induced labor: effects of pitocin, 209n.32; Karmel's experience, 47; Kitzinger's report, 141; Lang's observation, 160
*Immaculate Deception* (Arms), 174
*Implementing Family-Centered Maternity Care with a Central Nursery* (Haire and Haire), 114-115
Infant care advice: American reliance on experts, 75-77; concerning breastfeeding, 71-72, 76; during early 20th century, 76-77; modern conflicts, 94-95; theory of permissivness, 78
Infant Formula Action Coalition (INFACT), 72-74
Infant formula controversy, 72-74; ICEA campaign for regulating U.S. industry in hospitals, 75; report on Third World women's need to supplement breastmilk, 200n.14. *See also* summer illness
Infant mortality: decline in 20th century, 119-120; decline in nurse-midwifery services, 11-12, 13, 178; statistics corrected for age groups, 205n.42; relationship of decline to use of electronic monitor, 119-121; rates in minority communities, 175, 177. *See also* summer illness; bottle baby disease; risks in childbirth, infant
Infants' milk stations, early 20th century, 71
Informed Homebirth, 188
Institute of Feminine Arts, Santa Cruz, 187-188
International Childbirth Education Association (ICEA): and breastfeeding, 75, 96; and divorce, 68; founding and early membership, 25, 62-63, 78; subcommittee on home birth, 97; 1968 conference, 65. *See also* reform movement in childbirth

International Federation of Obstetrician Gynecologists, 116
Intervention in birth processes, vii; in history of obstetrics, 101-107; favored by social and legal concerns, 107-108. *See also* obstetrics profession; obstetrics technology; social forces affecting childbirth

Jackson, Edith, 32
Jackson, Molly, 155
Jacobson, Gregory C., 167
Jerliffe, Derrick B., 89
*Journal of the American Medical Association,* 131, 153
*Journal of Pediatrics,* 80

Karmel, Marjorie, 52; co-founding ASPO with Bing, 48-51; death, 50-51; Lamaze birth in Paris, 42-43; Lamaze birth in New York, 45-47
Keegan, Kirk A., Jr., 206n.58
Kennell, Johm, 140, 159
Kerwin, Mary Ann, 88
Kitzinger, Sheila, ix, 189; episiotomy studies, 142; induced labor studies, 141; life and work, 133-142; psychosexual method, 136-137; publications 141; "splendid ritual," 139-140
Klaus, Marshall, 94, 140, 159
Krisman, Michael, 177
Kushner, Rose, 193

Labor methods. *See* Bradley; Gamper; Lamaze; modified Lamaze; psychoprophylaxis; psychosexual; Read methods
*Ladies Home Journal,* 3, 53, 127; "Cruelty on the Maternity Wards," x, 55-57; history of ACE, 61; "Tell Me, Doctor," 30; "Why Should Mothers Die?" 6-9
La Leche League International (LLLI), 98, 113, 191; founding and growth, 87-91; and maternal guilt, 93-94; relationship to medical profession, 89-90; 94-95; and sexual aspects of breastfeeding, 90-91; and weaning, 92; and working mothers, 95-97. *See also* breastfeeding
*La Leche League Love Story,* 88
Lamaze. Fernand, 42-44
Lamaze method, vii, viii, 189; influence on American culture, 52; origin and growth, 42-44 *See also* ASPO; Bing;

Karmel; psychoprophylaxis
Lang, Raven, viii, 174, 186, 195; *Birth Book*, 158, 163-164; life and work 156-164; home birth, 186-187; and Santa Cruz Birth Center 161-163; and spiritual healing, 187-188
Larsen, Virginia, 12, 63, 85, 127; and early parent-education in Seattle, 33; and founding of ACE, 61
Lay interference, principle of, 211n.75
Leboyer birth, 189
Leboyer, Frederick, 4-5, 164
Lempke, Mary, 31-32
Lennon, Viola, 88
Lerner, Gerda, x-xi, 189
Levey, Julius, 154
Levy, Judith, 185
Liebeskind, Doreen, 117; ultrasound research, 127-130
Lithotomy position, 5-6
Litigation: advocated in DCA hearings, 179; as tool of childbirth reformers, 179-182, 193, 203n.28; used by medical profession to restrict midwives, 172-173; as way of protecting midwives and home births, 98. *See also* court cases; malpractice crisis
Llaminaria tents, 203n.15
Lobenstine Midwifery Clinic, 13. *See also* nurse-midwives
Lokas, Kitti, 161
Lubic, Ruth, 183
Lumley, Judith, 93, 121, 124

Madera nurse-midwife project, 178
*Making Love During Pregnancy* (Bing), 51
*Malleus Maleficarum* (Kramer and Sprenger), 147
Malpractice crisis of 1970s, 107-108; and increased cesarean rate, 127; as perceived by medical and legal profession, 108, 181, 203n.28 *See also* litigation
Mann, Rosemary J., 182-183
March of Dimes 1982 symposium, evaluation of ultrasound, 128, 130-131
Marieskind, Helen I., 117, 123-127
Martin, W. Darrell, 179-180
*Maternal Emotions* (Newton), 80
Maternal mortality: De Kruif 1936 series, "Why Should Mothers Die?", 6-9; current rate among poor and minority women, 175, 177; past rates, 4, 105; record of maternal deaths from alternative and midwife services,

9, 11, 13, 153-154, 178
*Maternité Du Métallurgiste*, 44
Maternity Center Association (MCA), 61, 186; MCA Childbearing Center, 183-184; and formation of ICEA, 62; history of, 12-14; and nurse-midwife training, 13-14; and sponsorship Yale Program, 31, 33
Maxwell Street Dispensary, 6
*McCalls's*, 100-101
McFalls, Joseph, 95
Mead, Margaret, 63; involvement with childbirth reform, 83
"Meddlesome Midwifery," 4, 103
Medi-Cal, 169
Medical-industrial alliance, 107-108; affect on health care, 175, 191
Medical profession: and La Leche League, 95; and lay interference, 211n.75; opposition to other practitioners, 180-181, 192-193, 209n.26; as regarded by early childbirth reformers, 61-62. *See also* obstetrical profession
Medical technology, 116, 131. *See also* obstetrical technology
Mehl, Louis, 162
Melendy, Mary Ries, vii, 14-15
Mendelsohn, Robert, 91
Mendenhall, Dorothy Reed, 4, 114
Midwest Parentcraft Center, 24-26
*The Midwife* (Courter), 194
Midwifery advocates, 62, 189, 192; DCA final report, 177-178
Midwives: alliance with nurse-midwives 194-195; California arrests, 164-172, 210n.49; history of 146-149, 207-208n.2; competition with male doctors, 149-150; new-age, 62, 155-156, 186, 189; versus medical profession, 153-155, 161, 173, 177-178, 192. *See* Chapter Five
Midwives Association of North America (MANA) 194-195
Miller, C. Arden, 116
Miller, Harold W., 21-23
Miller, John, 106
Modified Lamaze (Hazell) 64-65
Moen, Lynn, 96
Moggach, Debora, 133-134
Montagu, Ashley, 62, 63, 76, 78, 83; criticism of hospital births, 52-53
*Mother Earth News*, 98
Mothering: darker aspects, 93-94; hampered by hospital birth, 140; instinctive response, 158-159; L.L.L.I.

view, 89, 90, 92; qualities needed, 87; traditional lore, 78, 87. *See also* bonding; infant care advice

Mother's milk: rediscovered, 89-90; search for substitutes, 70

"Mothers and Outlaws," (Hunter), 172

*Ms*, 92

Murdough, Sister Angela, 194

Murphy, J.R., EFM studies, 204n.37

*Naissance* (Hommel), 48

*Nation*, 3

National Association of Childbearing Centers, 210n.82

National Association of Parents and Professionals for Safe Alternatives Childbirth (NAPSAC), 97-98, 170, 172, 185, 194

National Childbirth Trust, 133, 134, 141, 142

National Institute for Neurological and Communicative Disorders and Stroke, 117, 121

National Women's Health Network, ix, 123, 144

Native birth rituals, 138

Natural childbirth: at Chicago Maternity Center, 9; conflicting response from doctors, 40-41; early observations, 14-15; *McCall's* survey of doctors, 100-101; papal approval, 44-45. *See also* labor methods

Neonatal intensive care units, 175, 176-177

Nihill, Elizabeth, 149-150

Nestlé Company and infant formula regulations, 72-74

New Life Center, 182

*The New York Times*, 1-2

Newland, Kathleen, 120

Newell, Edith, 85

*Newsweek*, 100

Newton, Michael, 78

Newton, Niles, ix; cultural and biological requirements for motherhood, 86-87; life and work, 78-87; sensual aspects of breastfeeding and reproduction, 80-81, 91, 136; status of mothers, 191; support for working mothers, 95, 96

Nielsen, Gertrude, 1-3

"Nipple Pain and Nipple Damage," (Newton), 80

Northwestern University, 78; and demise of CMC, 9

Nurse Midwifery Associates, 179

Nurse-midwives: achievements, 11-12, 178; alliance with lay midwives, 194-195; modern concepts, 53, 155, 168; struggle to obtain back-up, insurance payments, and hospital privileges, 178-182, 211n.72; use of legal avenues for obtaining right to practice, 180-182; training, 13, 68. *See also* midwives

Nurses, 56, 203n.20

Oakley, Ann, 191

O'Brien, William, 130

Obstetrical training. *See* physician training

Obstetrical drugs. *See* drugs in labor and delivery

Obstetrical technology: recent advances 100, 107, 190-191; costs, 175-177; criticism, 120, 183-184; opposition in Britain, 132-133. *See also* cesarean section; electronic fetal monitoring; forceps; induced labor; intervention; medical-industrial alliance; ultrasound; version

*Obstetrics and Gynecology in America: A History* (Speert), 203nn.10-14, 16, 18

Obstetrics profession: criticism of various labor methods, 40-41, 49-50; history of, 101-106; discarded interventions of past, 131-132; opposition to midwives and nurse-midwives, 153-154, 161, 168; refusal of California obstetricians to take certain patients, 161, 169. *See also* control of birth; intervention

*Our Bodies, Ourselves*, (Boston Women's Health Book Collective), 194

"Ovarian mayhem," 104 *See also* gynecological surgery

Oxytocin, 81; role in let-down reflex, 79-80

Pain in childbirth: and anesthetic drugs, 2-3, 16, 150; as altered by natural and prepared labor techniques, 15, 40-41, 42-44, 136-137

Palmer, Harriet, 181

Paré, Ambrois, 101

Parent and Child Association, 61

*Pathology of the Fetus and Infant*, (Potter), 170

Patton, Edith, 127

Paukert, Sheryle, 115

Pavlovian theories, 43, 138

Peterson, David, 170

Physician training, 115, 175-176, 190-191
"Pit drip," 160. *See also* induced labor
Place of birth. *See* control of birth; home birth
Popular Health Movement, 150-151. *See also* consumers' rights in birth
Potter, Edith, 170-171
Poverty: as affecting health services, 175-177; as an element in bottle baby disease, 74-75; record of nurse-midwife and alternative birth services for poor women, 7, 178
Practitioners, mid-level and alternative in health professions, 192-193
*Preparation for the Heirminded* (Gamper), 25
Privor, David, 207n.92
Pryor, Karen, 54, 93
Psychoprophylaxis, 44, 46. *See also* Lamaze method
Psychosexual theory of childbirth (Kitzinger), 136-137. *See also* maternal mortality
Puerperal fever, 7-8. *See also* maternal mortality

Rakowitz, Elly, 48, 50, 52; founding of ASPO, 94
Raphael, Dana, 93; history of bottlefeeding, 69, 78; supplementary feedings study, 200n.14
Rawlins, Carolyn Mann, 63, 85; early childbirth educator, 191
Read, Grantly, Dick-, 31, 85; origin of theories on birth, 14-17. *See also* Read Method
Read, Jessica, 16
Read Method, vii; contrast with Lamaze method, 42-43; early reaction in U.S., 17-18; employed by Bing, 36-37; contribution to MCA and Yale Program, 31-32, 61. *See also* Gamper method; natural childbirth
*The Red Book* (Bing and Karmel), 50
*Redbook*, x, 63
Reform movement in childbirth: advances threatened by technology, 190; assessment of gains and failures, 106, 184, 185, 190; early attitude toward medical profession, 48-49, 62-63. *See also* litigation; organizations: ACE, ASPO, ICEA, NAPSAC
*Relax, Here's Your Baby* (Gamper), 25
Rennert, Zila, 49
Research, medical: assessment of current state, 115-116, concerning fetal distress, 204n.37; controversy over

clinical trials, 120-121, 205n.43. *See also* counterstream research
*Resource Guide on Maternal Health and Childbirth*, 144
Rhodes, Phillip, 131-132
Ribble, Margaret, 78
Rich, Adrienne, xi, 137, 191-192
Richardson, Frank Howard, 70, 77
Richwald, Gary, 131; function of ABCs, 183
Risks in childbirth, infant: due to holding back birth, 56-57; due to cesarean prematurity, 205n.54; due to effects of obstetric drugs, 32-33, 52, 121-123; fetal distress, 204n.37; reduced by prenatal care, 13. *See also* Counterstream research, Chapter Four
Risks in childbirth, maternal: as exacerbated by hospital routine, 53. *See also* cesarean section; episiotomy; induced labor
Romalis, Shelly, 142-143
Rothman, Barbara Katz, 88, 90, 191
Rubin, Reva: bonding theories, 94, 209n.31

Safety in childbirth: as concept, 99, 122-123. *See also* risks in childbirth
Safford, Henry B., 30, 57
Salisbury, Lois, 75
Santa Cruz Birth Center, California, 156, 161-167, 187; 1972 symposium, 162-163
Sawyer, Blackwell, 18
Scully, Diane, 86, 191
Segal, Benjamin, 48
Seiden, Anne, 95
Sellers, Lea, 132
Semmelweis, Ignatz, 7-8, 16
Sexual aspects of childbirth: breastfeeding, 90-93; episiotomy, 142-143; Bing on intercourse during pregnancy, 51; Kitzinger's psychosexual labor method, 136-137; Newton's theories, 80-81
Shauf, Victoria, 95
Shaw, Nancy Stoller, 191
Shearer, Beth, 126
Shearer, Madeleine, 178, 181; and routine intervention, 108-109
"Shelf and bulge" breathing, 25
Sheppard-Towner Bill, 154, 209n.26
Shorter, Edward, 207-208n.2
*Silent Knife: Cesarean Prevention and Vaginal Birth after Cesarean* (Cohen and Estner), 126

Simpson, James, 16
Sims, J. Marion, 104
*Six Practical Lessons for an Easier Childbirth* (Bing), 51
Sizemore, Susan, 179-180
Smith, Anthony, 147-148
Social forces affecting childbirth: contemporary movements favoring reform, 106, 155, 192-193; trends favoring obstetrical intervention, 2-3, 29-30, 76, 107-108
Solomon, Merilyn, 95
*Some Women's Experience of Episiotomy* (Kitzinger), 142
*Some Women's Experience of Induced Labor* (Kitzinger), 141
Speert, Harold, 124
*Spiritual Midwifery* (Gaskin), 184
"Splendid Ritual," (Kitzinger) 139-140
Spock, Benjamin, 78
Starr, Paul, 208-209n.13
Stewart, David, 97, 155, 194, 204-205n.42
Stewart, Lee, 97, 194
Stratmeyer, M.E., 130
Summer illness-1900s, 71-72. *See also* bottle baby disease; infant mortality
Summerhayes, Liz, 180
Swenson, Norma, vii, 190, 194

Tarpening, Rosalie, 168-172
Technology. *See* obstetrical technology
"Tell Me, Doctor" (Safford), 30
Thacker, Stephen: review of EFM research, 117-121
*Thank You, Doctor Lamaze* (Karmel), 48, 50
"Theft of Childbirth" (Rich), 137
Third World: infant formula controversy, 72-74; infant and maternal welfare in minority communities, 175, 177
Thompson, James R., 120
Thoms, Herbert, and Yale Program, 31-32
Thomson, Samuel, 151
Tompson, Marian, 88, 98
Touch Relaxation (Kitzinger), 137
Tucker, Beatrice: Director of Chicago Maternity Center, 6-10
Twilight Sleep, 2. *See also* drugs in labor and delivery

Ullman, Dana, 192
Ultrasound: development and controversies over use, 127-131

Valvanne, Leena, 109
Vanderbilt, Anne, 112
VBAC (vaginal birth after cesarean), 126
Vellay, Pierre, 46, 47, 49, 65
Version: external, 105, 203n.18; internal: an ancient maneuver, 101; use in 19th and 20th centuries, 103, 105. *See also* breech presentation
Victoria, Queen: use of anesthesia for birth, 3, 16
Villa, Graciella and baby, 169-171
Virgil, Cherilee, 167
"Viva's Breastfeeding Caper" (Viva), 92-93

Wagner, Betty, 88, 89
Walker, Jeanine, 164, 174
Watson, John B.: early 20th century infant care advice, 76-77
*A Way to Natural Childbirth* (Heardman), 31
Weaning, 93-94; the older child, 92
Weight gain in pregnancy, 131
Wertman, Judith, 70
Wertz, Dorothy C. and Wertz, Richard W., 5-6
Wessel, Helen, 106, 203n.23
Wet nurses, 69-70
White, Gregory, 88-89, 98
White, Mary, 88, 97
Wilf, Ruth, 185-186
Williams, John Whitridge, 5
Wilson, Sloan, 53-54
Witchcraze, European: midwives victims of persecution, 146-147; conflicting theories on origin, 208n.3
Withrow, Genna, 194
*Woman in Residence* (Harrison), 143
Women: attendants for other women in birth, 146-147; categorized by doctors in terms of interest in natural childbirth, 40-41; in health professions, 115, 190-191, 212n.5; invalidism in 19th century, 152; as obstetrical and gynecological patients, 30-31, 86-87, 212n.8; qualities necessary for motherhood, 86-87; recovery of history, vii, xi; status post World War II, 29; supporters of early welfare programs 12, 154, 209n.26. *See also* feminism
Women, Infants, and Children federal program (WIC), 120
Women's health movement, 144, 193, 194

Woods, Michael, 108, 123
World Health Organization (WHO), 80;
  and infant formula guidelines, 74-75

Yale Program for Prepared Childbirth,
  31-32, 41
Younger, Janet B., 94

# ABOUT THE AUTHORS

Margot Edwards became an activist in the women's health movement after working as a hospital nurse. She has been a childbirth educator for seventeen years and has written extensively on the politics and process of birth. Her professional commitments have included working with ICEA, NAPSAC and the periodical BIRTH: ISSUES IN PERINATAL CARE. She lives with her husband David. Between them, they have six children. Her current interests include whitewater canoeing, singing and promoting midwifery.

Mary Waldorf worked with the Actor's Workshop in San Francisco for ten years as an actress-technician. She was director and finally a playwright in their children's theater. She has published two novels for young children as well as a children's play. Presently, she is at work on an adult historical novel. Her involvement in the childbirth movement springs from her own experiences giving birth and has developed through her collaborative work with Margot Edwards. She is the mother of two children and four stepchildren.

*Other books published by The Crossing Press which may be of particular interest:*

**NATURAL BIRTH poems by Toi Derricotte**

**THE WHOLE BIRTH CATALOG: A SOURCEBOOK FOR CHOICES IN CHILDBIRTH edited by Janet Isaacs Ashford**

Our complete catalog of publications is available on request. Please write to us at The Crossing Press, Main Street, Trumansburg, New York 14886.